# THE COMPREHENSIVE GUIDE TO GLYCEMIC INDEX AND GLYCEMIC LOAD COUNTERS WITH 3500+ FOODS

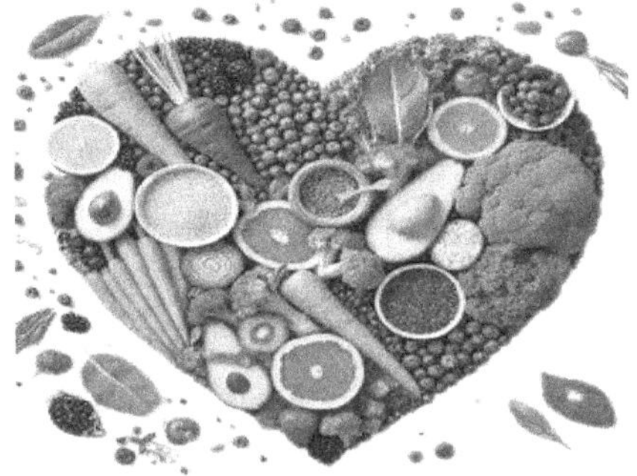

## Unlocking the Low Glycemic Diets Secrets to Optimal Health and Weight Management Through Informed Dietary Choices

## Luisa pace

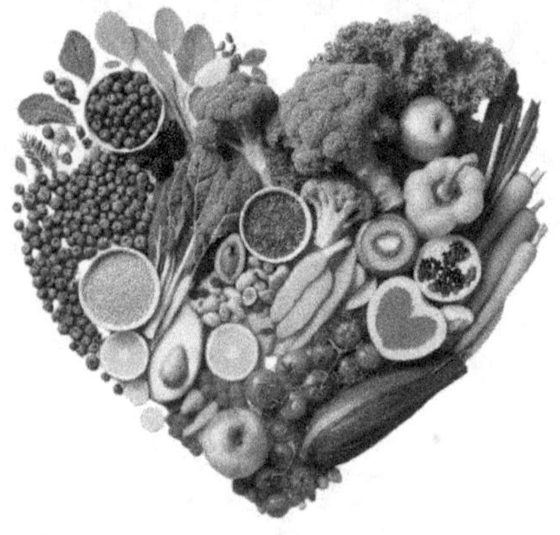

# TABLE OF CONTENTS

# INTRODUCTION

The Glycemic Index (GI) is a crucial concept in nutrition that classifies carbohydrate-containing foods based on their impact on blood sugar levels. It provides a numerical ranking to these foods, indicating how quickly or slowly they cause a spike in blood glucose after consumption. The scale ranges from 0 to 100, with higher values signifying a faster and greater increase in blood sugar.

## Understanding the Glycemic Index

The GI is a scale that measures how rapidly carbohydrates are converted into glucose and absorbed into the bloodstream.

**Foods are categorized into three main groups:**

1. Low-GI (55 and below): These foods release glucose slowly, leading to a gradual and sustained increase in blood sugar levels.
2. Moderate-GI (56-69): These foods cause a moderate rise in blood glucose.
3. High-GI (70 and above): These foods result in a rapid spike in blood sugar levels.
4. The concept was originally developed to help individuals with diabetes manage their blood sugar levels, but it has since gained popularity for its relevance to weight management and overall health.

## Importance of the Glycemic Index

1. Blood Sugar Control: For individuals with diabetes, understanding the GI of foods is vital for maintaining stable blood sugar levels and preventing extreme highs and lows.
2. Weight Management: The GI is also a valuable tool for those looking to manage or lose weight. Low-GI foods often provide longer-lasting energy, reducing the likelihood of cravings and overeating.
3. Energy Levels: Choosing foods with a lower GI can help sustain energy levels throughout the day, preventing the energy crashes associated with high-GI foods.
4. Athletic Performance: Athletes can use the GI to optimize their carbohydrate intake for sustained energy during endurance activities.

## Factors Influencing Glycemic Response

1. Fiber Content: Foods high in fiber tend to have a lower GI because fiber slows down the digestion and absorption of carbohydrates.
2. Food Processing: Highly processed foods often have a higher GI compared to whole, minimally processed foods.
3. Fat and Protein Content: The presence of fats and proteins can lower the overall GI of a meal by slowing down the digestion and absorption of carbohydrates.

Understanding the Glycemic Index (GI) is of paramount importance in unraveling the intricacies of carbohydrate metabolism and its profound impact on overall health. Here's a detailed exploration of the significance of GI in understanding carbohydrates:

**Blood Sugar Regulation:**
1. Carbohydrates are the primary macronutrient responsible for elevating blood sugar levels. The GI provides a systematic approach to evaluating how different carbohydrates affect blood glucose levels.
2. High-GI carbohydrates lead to a rapid spike in blood sugar, triggering an equally rapid insulin response to lower glucose levels. This can be problematic for individuals with diabetes or insulin resistance.

**Diabetes Management:**
1. For individuals with diabetes, maintaining stable blood sugar levels is a critical aspect of disease management. The GI assists in identifying and selecting low-GI carbohydrates, which release glucose more slowly, preventing sudden spikes in blood sugar.
2. Incorporating low-GI foods can contribute to better glycemic control, reducing the need for insulin or other diabetes medications.

**Energy Levels and Satiety:**
1. Carbohydrates are a primary source of energy for the body. Choosing low-GI carbohydrates provides a more sustained release of glucose, offering a steady supply of energy over an extended period.
2. Low-GI foods also contribute to a feeling of fullness and satiety, reducing the likelihood of overeating and promoting weight management.

**Weight Management:**
1. The GI is a valuable tool for individuals aiming to manage or lose weight. High-GI foods can lead to rapid increases and subsequent crashes in blood sugar levels, often resulting in increased hunger and cravings.
2. Opting for low-GI carbohydrates can help control appetite, making it easier to adhere to a calorie-controlled diet.

**Physical Performance:**
1. Athletes and individuals engaged in regular physical activity can benefit from understanding the GI of carbohydrates. Consuming low-GI foods before and during endurance activities provides a sustained energy release, enhancing performance and delaying fatigue.

**Chronic Disease Prevention:**

- Research suggests that a diet based on low-GI foods may be associated with a reduced risk of chronic diseases, including cardiovascular disease and certain types of cancer.
- Low-GI diets are often rich in fiber, vitamins, and minerals, contributing to overall health and well-being.

## How GI Affects Blood Sugar Levels

**Rate of Glucose Absorption:**

- The GI categorizes carbohydrates based on how quickly they are converted into glucose and absorbed into the bloodstream. High-GI foods lead to a rapid surge in blood sugar, while low-GI foods result in a slower, more gradual increase.

**Insulin Response:**

- When blood sugar levels rise, the body releases insulin to facilitate the uptake of glucose by cells for energy or storage. High-GI foods prompt a rapid and often elevated insulin response to counteract the sudden increase in blood glucose.
- Consistently high insulin levels, as seen with frequent consumption of high-GI foods, can contribute to insulin resistance over time.

**Blood Sugar Peaks and Crashes:**

- High-GI foods can cause a sharp spike in blood sugar, followed by a rapid decline. This rollercoaster effect can lead to feelings of fatigue, irritability, and increased hunger shortly after consuming high-GI meals.
- On the other hand, low-GI foods provide a more sustained release of glucose, promoting stable blood sugar levels and preventing drastic peaks and crashes.

**Glycemic Load:**

- While the GI indicates the quality of carbohydrates, the Glycemic Load (GL) considers both the quality and quantity of carbohydrates in a specific serving. It provides a more accurate assessment of a food's impact on blood sugar.
- Foods with a low GI may still have a significant impact on blood sugar if consumed in large quantities, highlighting the importance of portion control.

**Impact on Diabetes Management:**

- Individuals with diabetes, in particular, can benefit from understanding how GI affects blood sugar levels. Low-GI foods are recommended to help maintain stable blood glucose, reducing the risk of hyperglycemia and the need for excessive insulin or medication.

- Managing the overall GI of meals is a key strategy in diabetes self-care, contributing to long-term glycemic control.

**Weight Management:**
- The impact of GI on blood sugar levels is closely linked to appetite regulation. High-GI foods may lead to increased hunger shortly after consumption, potentially contributing to overeating and weight gain.
- Choosing low-GI options can help control appetite, making it easier to manage calorie intake and support weight management goals.

Understanding the physiology of digestion and blood sugar regulation is essential for grasping how the body processes carbohydrates and maintains glucose levels within a narrow range. Here's an in-depth exploration of these processes:

**Carbohydrate Digestion:**
- The journey begins in the mouth, where salivary enzymes start breaking down complex carbohydrates into simpler sugars, like maltose.
- As food travels to the stomach, gastric acid continues the breakdown process. However, carbohydrates are not fully digested in the stomach.

**Small Intestine Absorption:**
- The majority of carbohydrate digestion occurs in the small intestine. Pancreatic enzymes and enzymes from the lining of the small intestine break down complex sugars into glucose, fructose, and galactose.
- These simple sugars are then absorbed into the bloodstream through the walls of the small intestine.

**Blood Sugar Regulation:**
- Upon absorption, glucose enters the bloodstream, causing blood sugar levels to rise. This triggers the release of insulin from the pancreas.
- Insulin's Role: Insulin acts as a key that unlocks cells, allowing them to take up glucose for energy or storage. This process lowers blood sugar levels, preventing them from reaching dangerously high levels.
- Storage of Glucose: Excess glucose is stored in the liver and muscles as glycogen. When blood sugar levels drop, the pancreas releases glucagon, signaling the liver to convert glycogen back into glucose for energy.

**Hormonal Regulation:**
- Hormones play a critical role in blood sugar regulation. Insulin and glucagon work in tandem to maintain glucose homeostasis.
- Insulin: Secreted in response to elevated blood sugar, insulin facilitates glucose uptake by cells, promoting its conversion to energy or storage.
- Glucagon: Released when blood sugar levels decrease, glucagon stimulates the liver to release stored glucose, raising blood sugar levels.

**Glycemic Index Influence:**
- The concept of the Glycemic Index (GI) comes into play here. Foods with a high GI lead to a rapid spike in blood sugar, prompting a swift insulin

response. Conversely, low-GI foods cause a slower, more sustained increase in blood glucose, leading to a more controlled insulin release.

**Impact of Fiber:**
- Fiber, an indigestible carbohydrate, slows down the absorption of glucose. This moderates the rise in blood sugar, contributing to a more stable and sustained release of energy.
- High-fiber diets are often associated with improved blood sugar control and reduced risk of type 2 diabetes.

# CARBOHYDRATE METABOLISM

Carbohydrate metabolism is a complex and highly regulated process that plays a central role in providing energy for various physiological functions. Here's a comprehensive exploration of the stages and intricacies of carbohydrate metabolism:

**Glycolysis:**

- Initiation: Carbohydrate metabolism often begins with glycolysis, which takes place in the cytoplasm of cells. During this process, a glucose molecule is broken down into two molecules of pyruvate.
- Energy Production: Glycolysis generates a small amount of ATP (adenosine triphosphate) directly and contributes to the production of reducing equivalents (NADH), which are crucial for subsequent energy production.

**Aerobic Respiration:**

- Citric Acid Cycle (Krebs Cycle): If oxygen is present, pyruvate enters the mitochondria and undergoes the citric acid cycle. This cycle produces additional NADH and FADH2, which carry high-energy electrons for the next stage.
- Electron Transport Chain (ETC): High-energy electrons from NADH and FADH2 are transferred through a series of protein complexes in the inner mitochondrial membrane. This transfer generates a

proton gradient, driving ATP synthesis in a process known as oxidative phosphorylation.

**Anaerobic Respiration (Lactic Acid Fermentation):**
- In the absence of oxygen, pyruvate can be converted into lactate in the cytoplasm. This process helps regenerate NAD+, allowing glycolysis to continue in conditions where oxygen is limited.
- While less efficient in terms of ATP production compared to aerobic respiration, anaerobic respiration serves as a crucial energy-generating mechanism in situations of oxygen scarcity.

**Glycogen Synthesis and Breakdown:**
- Excess glucose not immediately needed for energy is stored as glycogen in the liver and muscles. Glycogen synthesis occurs when blood glucose levels are elevated.
- Glycogen can be broken down through glycogenolysis to release glucose into the bloodstream when energy demand is high or blood glucose levels are low.

**Glucose Homeostasis:**
- The liver plays a central role in maintaining glucose homeostasis. It can release glucose through gluconeogenesis (the synthesis of glucose from non-carbohydrate sources) during fasting or low-blood-sugar conditions.

- Insulin and glucagon, hormones released by the pancreas, regulate blood glucose levels. Insulin facilitates glucose uptake by cells, while glucagon stimulates the release of stored glucose.

**Conversion of Carbohydrates to Fat:**
- Excess glucose that is not used for energy or stored as glycogen can be converted into fat through lipogenesis. This process is primarily regulated by insulin.

**Dietary Fiber Influence:**
- While dietary fiber is not metabolized for energy, it plays a significant role in carbohydrate metabolism by slowing down the absorption of glucose. This moderates blood sugar levels and contributes to sustained energy release.

## Managing Diabetes with the Glycemic Index

Managing diabetes involves careful attention to dietary choices, and the Glycemic Index (GI) is a valuable tool in this regard. Here's an in-depth exploration of how individuals with diabetes can effectively utilize the GI to regulate blood sugar levels and overall health:

**Understanding Glycemic Index and Load:**
- Individuals with diabetes need to be mindful of how quickly different carbohydrates affect blood sugar. The GI measures this impact, categorizing

foods based on their ability to raise blood glucose
levels.

- Glycemic Load (GL), which considers both the
  quantity and quality of carbohydrates, is equally
  important. It provides a more accurate picture of a
  food's impact on blood sugar.

**Choosing Low-GI Foods:**

- Low-GI foods have a slower and more controlled
  impact on blood sugar levels. These include whole
  grains, legumes, fruits, and vegetables.
- Incorporating low-GI foods into the diet helps
  prevent sudden spikes in blood glucose, promoting
  stable levels throughout the day.

**Balancing Carbohydrates with Other Nutrients:**

- While focusing on the GI is essential, it's equally
  important to balance carbohydrates with proteins,
  healthy fats, and fiber. This combination helps
  slow down the absorption of glucose and provides
  a sustained release of energy.
- Including sources of lean protein and healthy fats
  with each meal can improve glycemic control.

**Meal Planning for Diabetes:**

- Creating well-balanced, low-GI meals is a key
  aspect of diabetes management. Planning meals
  that include a variety of nutrient-dense foods helps
  regulate blood sugar levels and supports overall
  health.

- Considering portion sizes is crucial to avoid overloading the body with carbohydrates, even if they are low-GI.

**Monitoring Blood Sugar Responses:**
- Regularly monitoring blood sugar levels allows individuals with diabetes to understand how different foods impact their glycemic response.
- This self-monitoring empowers individuals to make informed choices and tailor their diet to their unique needs.

**Snacking Wisely:**
- Smart snacking is essential for individuals with diabetes. Opting for low-GI snacks helps maintain consistent energy levels between meals.
- Combining carbohydrates with protein or healthy fats in snacks can further stabilize blood sugar.

**Educating on Glycemic Index:**
- Diabetes management involves education. Providing individuals with diabetes the knowledge and skills to understand and utilize the GI empowers them to take control of their diet and, consequently, their blood sugar levels.

**Collaboration with Healthcare Professionals:**
- Collaborating with healthcare professionals, including dietitians and diabetes educators, ensures a personalized and comprehensive approach to diabetes management.
- Healthcare professionals can assist in creating individualized meal plans that consider the GI, lifestyle factors, and personal preferences.

## Understanding Glycemic Load

Understanding Glycemic Load (GL) is essential for making more precise and practical dietary choices, particularly for individuals managing conditions like diabetes or those aiming for better blood sugar control. While the Glycemic Index (GI) provides information about how quickly a specific food raises blood sugar, the Glycemic Load combines this with the actual quantity of carbohydrates consumed. Here's a detailed exploration of Glycemic Load:

**Definition of Glycemic Load:**
- Glycemic Load is a more comprehensive measure than the Glycemic Index. It takes into account not only the quality of carbohydrates (as indicated by the GI) but also the quantity of carbohydrates in a specific serving of a particular food.
- It provides a more accurate representation of a food's impact on blood sugar levels, as it considers both the speed of glucose release and the total amount of glucose released.

## Calculation of Glycemic Load:

- The formula for calculating Glycemic Load is: GL = (GI x Carbohydrate content in grams per serving) / 100.
- It multiplies the food's GI by the amount of available carbohydrates (total carbohydrates minus fiber) in a standard serving and then divides by 100.

## Interpretation of Glycemic Load:

- Low GL (10 or less): Foods with a low GL have a minimal impact on blood sugar. They are often considered favorable choices for individuals looking to manage blood sugar levels or control their weight.
- Moderate GL (11-19): Foods with a moderate GL have a moderate impact on blood sugar. Including them in moderation can be part of a balanced diet.
- High GL (20 or more): Foods with a high GL can cause a more significant spike in blood sugar. It's advisable to consume high-GL foods in moderation, especially for individuals with diabetes or insulin resistance.

## Practical Application:

- Choosing foods with a lower Glycemic Load helps individuals select options that are less likely to cause rapid fluctuations in blood sugar levels.
- For example, watermelon has a high GI, but its Glycemic Load per serving is relatively low

because it contains a small amount of carbohydrates per serving. This means that the impact on blood sugar is less than one might expect based solely on the GI.

**Combining GI and GL:**
- While the Glycemic Index is a valuable tool, it doesn't consider the quantity of carbohydrates in a serving. By combining GI and GL, individuals can make more nuanced decisions about their carbohydrate intake.
- For instance, a food with a high GI may have a lower impact on blood sugar if the serving size is small, resulting in a lower Glycemic Load.

**Influence on Meal Planning:**
- Understanding Glycemic Load is particularly useful in meal planning. By considering both the quality and quantity of carbohydrates, individuals can create well-balanced meals that support stable blood sugar levels and sustained energy throughout the day.

Weight management and the Glycemic Index (GI) are closely linked, as understanding how different carbohydrates affect blood sugar levels can play a pivotal role in achieving and maintaining a healthy weight. Here's a detailed exploration of the connection between weight management and the Glycemic Index:

**Role of Blood Sugar in Weight Management:**
- Blood sugar levels influence hunger, energy levels, and the body's storage of fat. Rapid spikes and crashes in blood sugar, often associated with high-GI foods, can lead to increased cravings and overeating.
- Stable blood sugar levels, achievable through the consumption of low-GI foods, contribute to better appetite control and may assist in weight management efforts.

**Satiety and Low-GI Foods:**
- Low-GI foods, which release glucose more slowly, contribute to a feeling of fullness and satiety. This sensation can help individuals consume fewer calories overall, making it easier to adhere to a calorie-controlled diet.
- Including low-GI foods in meals can promote satisfaction and reduce the likelihood of snacking on high-calorie, low-nutrient options.

**Preventing Overeating:**
- High-GI foods can trigger a cycle of overeating by causing rapid increases and subsequent drops in blood sugar. This often leads to increased hunger and cravings for more high-GI foods.
- Choosing low-GI options can break this cycle, providing a more sustained release of energy and reducing the urge to overeat.

**Managing Insulin Response:**
- High-GI foods prompt a rapid insulin response to lower elevated blood sugar levels. Consistently elevated insulin levels are associated with weight gain and insulin resistance.
- Consuming low-GI foods can help manage insulin response, potentially reducing the risk of insulin resistance and promoting a healthier weight.

**Energy Balance:**
- Weight management is fundamentally about maintaining a balance between calorie intake and expenditure. While the GI itself does not dictate the calorie content of foods, choosing low-GI options can support a more balanced and sustainable approach to weight control.
- Low-GI foods often provide longer-lasting energy, reducing the need for frequent snacking and helping individuals maintain an overall lower calorie intake.

**Physical Performance and Weight Loss:**

- For individuals engaging in physical activity for weight loss, incorporating low-GI foods into their diet can be beneficial. These foods provide sustained energy during workouts and aid in post-exercise recovery.
- The sustained energy release from low-GI foods can support consistent exercise patterns, contributing to long-term weight management.

**Long-Term Sustainability:**

- Diets based on low-GI principles are often more sustainable in the long term. They emphasize whole, nutrient-dense foods that provide essential vitamins and minerals, promoting overall health and well-being.
- Sustainable weight management involves adopting dietary patterns that can be maintained over time, and low-GI foods contribute to this by providing a balanced and satisfying approach to eating.

## Role of GI in Hunger and Satiety

The Glycemic Index (GI) plays a crucial role in regulating hunger and satiety, influencing how individuals perceive and respond to the feeling of fullness. Understanding this role is key to making informed dietary choices and managing appetite effectively. Here's a detailed exploration of the role of GI in hunger and satiety:

**Blood Sugar Fluctuations and Hunger:**

- High-GI foods cause a rapid spike in blood sugar levels, followed by a quick decline. This fluctuation can trigger feelings of hunger shortly after consuming such foods.
- Rapid changes in blood sugar prompt the release of hunger hormones, signaling to the body that it needs more fuel. This can lead to increased cravings and a higher likelihood of overeating.

**Sustained Energy Release:**

- Low-GI foods release glucose into the bloodstream more gradually. This results in a slower, more sustained energy release over time.
- The steady availability of energy helps maintain blood sugar levels within a normal range, reducing the frequency and intensity of hunger signals.

**Effect on Ghrelin and Leptin:**

- Ghrelin is known as the "hunger hormone" because it stimulates appetite. High-GI foods can increase ghrelin levels, contributing to feelings of hunger.
- Leptin, on the other hand, is the "satiety hormone" that signals fullness to the brain. Low-GI foods may help maintain optimal leptin levels, promoting a greater sense of satiety.

**Appetite Control:**
- Including low-GI foods in meals promotes better appetite control. These foods contribute to a feeling of fullness and satisfaction, reducing the likelihood of snacking on high-calorie, low-nutrient options.
- Choosing a diet rich in low-GI foods may assist in managing overall calorie intake, making it easier for individuals to adhere to weight management goals.

**Impact on Meal Timing:**
- Consuming low-GI foods can help individuals maintain stable energy levels between meals. This reduces the need for frequent snacking, particularly on foods that are high in sugar and provide only temporary relief from hunger.
- Stable energy levels throughout the day contribute to a more regular eating pattern and can aid in weight management.

**Combination with Fiber and Nutrients:**
- Low-GI foods are often rich in fiber, which adds bulk to meals and promotes a feeling of fullness. Fiber also slows down the digestion and absorption of carbohydrates, contributing to sustained satiety.
- Nutrient-dense low-GI foods provide essential vitamins and minerals, supporting overall health while helping control hunger.

**Role in Weight Management:**

- The relationship between GI, hunger, and satiety is pivotal in weight management. Consuming a diet that includes more low-GI foods helps individuals control their appetite, leading to a more balanced and sustainable approach to weight loss or maintenance.
- Low-GI diets are associated with better adherence over the long term, contributing to successful weight management.

## Using GI to Make Informed Food Choices for Weight Loss

Leveraging the Glycemic Index (GI) to make informed food choices is a strategic approach for individuals aiming for weight loss. By understanding how different carbohydrates affect blood sugar levels and hunger, one can create a diet that promotes sustained energy and better appetite control. Here's a detailed exploration of using GI for weight loss:

**Choosing Low-GI Foods:**

- Low-GI foods release glucose slowly, providing a more sustained and steady source of energy. Prioritize these foods in your diet to avoid the rapid spikes and crashes in blood sugar associated with high-GI options.
- Examples of low-GI foods include whole grains, legumes, fruits, vegetables, and nuts.

**Prioritizing Fiber-Rich Foods:**

- Many low-GI foods are also rich in dietary fiber, which contributes to feelings of fullness and satiety. Fiber adds bulk to meals, slowing down the digestion and absorption of carbohydrates.
- Foods such as whole grains, fruits, vegetables, and legumes are excellent sources of fiber.

**Balancing Macronutrients:**

- While focusing on the GI, it's essential to balance carbohydrates with proteins and healthy fats. Including protein and fats in meals helps stabilize blood sugar levels and promotes a feeling of fullness.
- Incorporate lean proteins, such as poultry, fish, beans, and tofu, and healthy fats, like avocados, nuts, and olive oil, into your meals.

**Understanding Portion Sizes:**

- While low-GI foods are beneficial, portion control remains crucial for weight loss. Be mindful of overall calorie intake and avoid overeating, even with low-GI options.
- Use appropriate serving sizes to create a balanced and calorie-controlled diet.

**Limiting Highly Processed Foods:**

- Highly processed foods often have a higher GI due to the refining and stripping of fiber. These foods

can contribute to rapid spikes in blood sugar and increased cravings.
- Choose whole, minimally processed foods whenever possible to support weight loss goals.

## Incorporating Variety:
- Diversify your diet by including a variety of low-GI foods. This ensures a broad spectrum of nutrients and flavors, making the diet more enjoyable and sustainable.
- Experiment with different grains, fruits, and vegetables to keep meals interesting and satisfying.

## Smart Snacking with Low-GI Options:
- Snacking on low-GI foods can help control hunger between meals. Opt for snacks that combine carbohydrates with protein or healthy fats to maintain a stable blood sugar level.
- Examples of low-GI snacks include Greek yogurt with berries, apple slices with nut butter, or raw vegetables with hummus.

## Monitoring and Adjusting:
- Regularly monitor your response to different foods by paying attention to hunger levels and energy throughout the day. Adjust your diet as needed to find a balance that supports weight loss and overall well-being.

- Keep a food diary or use apps that track your meals to identify patterns and make informed adjustments.

**Collaborating with Healthcare Professionals:**
- Consult with healthcare professionals, such as dietitians or nutritionists, for personalized advice tailored to your specific needs and health conditions.
- Professional guidance ensures that your weight loss strategy aligns with your overall health goals and is sustainable in the long term.

## Principles and tips for low glycemic eating

**Understand the Glycemic Index (GI):**
Familiarize yourself with the GI values of various foods. Lower GI foods release glucose more slowly and have a gentler impact on blood sugar.

**Prioritize Whole Grains:**
Choose whole grains such as quinoa, brown rice, and oats over refined grains. Whole grains contain more fiber, contributing to a lower GI.

**Include Legumes:**
Legumes like lentils, chickpeas, and black beans are excellent sources of protein and fiber, making them low-GI choices that provide lasting satiety.

**Embrace Non-Starchy Vegetables:**
Load your plate with non-starchy vegetables like leafy greens, broccoli, and cauliflower. These are nutrient-dense, low in calories, and have a minimal impact on blood sugar.

**Opt for Lean Proteins:**
Choose lean protein sources such as poultry, fish, tofu, and legumes. Protein-rich foods help stabilize blood sugar and promote a feeling of fullness.

**Include Healthy Fats:**
Incorporate sources of healthy fats, like avocados, nuts, and olive oil. Fats slow down digestion, reducing the overall glycemic impact of a meal.

**Balanced Meals:**
Aim for balanced meals that include a combination of carbohydrates, proteins, and fats. This helps maintain stable blood sugar levels and provides sustained energy.

**Mindful Portion Control:**
Be mindful of portion sizes to manage overall calorie intake. Even low-GI foods can contribute to weight gain if consumed in excessive amounts.

**Choose Whole Fruits:**
Whole fruits, such as berries, apples, and pears, have a lower GI compared to fruit juices or processed fruit

products. The fiber content in whole fruits further moderates their glycemic impact.

**Avoid Sugary Beverages:**
Steer clear of sugary drinks and opt for water, herbal tea, or unsweetened beverages. Sugary drinks can lead to rapid spikes in blood sugar.

**Combine Foods Smartly:**
Pair high-GI foods with low-GI foods to create a balanced meal. Combining macronutrients helps mitigate the overall glycemic impact.

**Snack Wisely:**
Choose low-GI snacks such as Greek yogurt with berries, raw vegetables with hummus, or a handful of nuts. These snacks provide sustained energy and curb cravings.

**Read Food Labels:**
Check food labels for the carbohydrate content and choose products with lower total carbohydrates and higher fiber content.

*Cooking Methods Matter:*
Opt for cooking methods like steaming, roasting, or grilling instead of frying. These methods help retain nutrients and maintain the low-GI nature of foods.

**Include Fiber-Rich Foods:**
Fiber-rich foods, including whole grains, vegetables, and legumes, slow down the digestion of carbohydrates, promoting better blood sugar control.

**Be Cautious with Processed Foods:**
Limit the intake of highly processed foods, as they often have higher GI values due to reduced fiber content.

**Plan Balanced Meals:**
Plan your meals to include a variety of low-GI foods, ensuring a mix of nutrients and flavors for a satisfying and nutritious diet.

**Stay Hydrated:**
Drink plenty of water throughout the day. Proper hydration supports overall health and can help control appetite.

**Regular Physical Activity:**
Engage in regular physical activity, as exercise can enhance insulin sensitivity and improve blood sugar control.

**Consult with a Professional:**
If you have specific health concerns or dietary needs, consult with a healthcare professional or a registered dietitian for personalized guidance on low glycemic eating.

# Detailed food list to include in your low glycemic diet

A low glycemic diet emphasizes foods that have a minimal impact on blood sugar levels, promoting stable energy and better overall health. Here's a detailed list of foods to include in your low glycemic diet:

**Non-Starchy Vegetables:**
Include a variety of non-starchy vegetables such as leafy greens, broccoli, cauliflower, zucchini, bell peppers, and asparagus. These vegetables are rich in fiber and essential nutrients.

**Leafy Greens:**
Incorporate leafy greens like spinach, kale, and Swiss chard. These vegetables are low in carbohydrates and high in fiber, making them excellent choices for a low glycemic diet.

**Berries:**
Choose berries such as blueberries, strawberries, and raspberries. Berries are high in antioxidants and fiber, providing sweetness without a significant impact on blood sugar.

**Apples and Pears:**
Opt for whole apples and pears, which are lower in sugar compared to some other fruits. The fiber content helps slow down the digestion of carbohydrates.

**Legumes:**
Include legumes like lentils, chickpeas, black beans, and kidney beans. Legumes are rich in fiber and protein, offering sustained energy and promoting fullness.

**Quinoa:**
Quinoa is a versatile whole grain that is high in protein and fiber. It has a lower impact on blood sugar compared to refined grains.

**Brown Rice:**
Choose brown rice over white rice. Brown rice is a whole grain that retains its fiber content, providing a slower release of glucose.

**Oats:**
Opt for old-fashioned oats or steel-cut oats. Oats contain beta-glucans, a type of soluble fiber that supports stable blood sugar levels.

**Greek Yogurt:**
Greek yogurt is rich in protein and lower in carbohydrates compared to some other dairy products. Choose plain, unsweetened Greek yogurt to avoid added sugars.

**Nuts and Seeds:**
Include nuts such as almonds, walnuts, and pistachios, as well as seeds like chia seeds and flaxseeds. These are nutrient-dense snacks that provide healthy fats and protein.

**Avocados:**
Avocados are a great source of monounsaturated fats, which contribute to a feeling of fullness. They are low in carbohydrates and have a minimal impact on blood sugar.

**Sweet Potatoes:**
Choose sweet potatoes over white potatoes. Sweet potatoes have a lower glycemic index and are rich in fiber, vitamins, and minerals.

**Salmon and Other Fatty Fish:**
Fatty fish like salmon, mackerel, and trout provide omega-3 fatty acids and protein. Including these in your diet supports overall health and satiety.

**Eggs:**
Eggs are a protein-rich, low-carbohydrate option that can be included in various dishes. They provide essential amino acids and nutrients.

**Tofu and Tempeh:**
Tofu and tempeh are plant-based protein sources that can be included in vegetarian or plant-based low glycemic meals.

**Herbs and Spices:**
Use herbs and spices like cinnamon, turmeric, and ginger to add flavor without added sugars or high-GI condiments.

**Garlic and Onions:**
Garlic and onions add flavor to meals without significantly impacting blood sugar. They also offer various health benefits.

**Tea and Coffee:**
Unsweetened tea and black coffee can be consumed in moderation. These beverages are low in calories and don't contribute to blood sugar spikes.

**Mushrooms:**
Include mushrooms in your meals. They are low in carbohydrates and can add texture and flavor to various dishes.

**Cheese (in moderation):**
Choose cheese in moderation, focusing on varieties that are lower in fat. Cheese provides protein and can be a satisfying snack or addition to meals.

Avoiding high glycemic and inflammatory foods is crucial for promoting overall health, managing chronic conditions, and preventing inflammation-related issues. Here's a detailed discussion on why and how to avoid these foods:

**High Glycemic Foods:**

- High glycemic foods are those that cause a rapid spike in blood sugar levels. These foods include refined carbohydrates, sugary snacks, and processed foods.
- Rapid blood sugar spikes can contribute to insulin resistance, weight gain, and inflammation, which are associated with various health issues.

**Inflammatory Foods:**

- Inflammatory foods are those that promote inflammation in the body. These often include processed foods, excessive sugar, trans fats, and certain additives.
- Chronic inflammation is linked to conditions such as cardiovascular disease, diabetes, and autoimmune disorders.

# Reasons to Avoid High Glycemic and Inflammatory Foods

**Blood Sugar Regulation:**
High glycemic foods can lead to erratic blood sugar levels, increasing the risk of insulin resistance. Stable blood sugar is essential for overall health and energy balance.

**Inflammation Control:**
Avoiding inflammatory foods helps control chronic inflammation, reducing the risk of inflammatory conditions and promoting optimal immune function.

**Weight Management:**
High glycemic and inflammatory foods often contribute to weight gain. Avoiding these foods supports weight management efforts and reduces the risk of obesity-related inflammation.

**Energy Stability:**
Choosing low glycemic foods helps maintain stable energy levels throughout the day, preventing energy crashes and reducing the need for constant snacking.

**Refined Carbohydrates:**
Limit or avoid white bread, white rice, and other refined grains. Choose whole grains for a slower release of glucose.

**Processed Snacks:**
Snack foods like cookies, chips, and candies are often high in both refined carbohydrates and inflammatory additives. Opt for whole, minimally processed snacks.

**Sugary Beverages:**
Sugary drinks, including sodas and fruit juices, contribute to rapid blood sugar spikes. Choose water, herbal tea, or unsweetened alternatives.

**Trans Fats:**
Trans fats, often found in processed and fried foods, are known to promote inflammation. Check labels and avoid products with trans fats.

**Excessive Sweets:**
Limit your intake of cakes, pastries, and other high-sugar desserts. Choose healthier alternatives with natural sweeteners in moderation.

**Processed Meats:**
Processed meats, like sausages and hot dogs, may contain additives linked to inflammation. Opt for lean, unprocessed protein sources.

**Fast Food:**
Fast food is often high in both refined carbohydrates and unhealthy fats. Choose home-cooked meals with fresh ingredients.

**Highly Processed Foods:**
Foods with long ingredient lists and artificial additives may contribute to inflammation. Focus on whole, single-ingredient foods.

**Excessive Alcohol:**
High alcohol consumption can contribute to inflammation. Consume alcohol in moderation or choose alternatives like red wine, which may have anti-inflammatory properties.

## Tips for Choosing Anti-Inflammatory Alternatives

**Load Up on Fruits and Vegetables:**
Colorful fruits and vegetables are rich in antioxidants and anti-inflammatory compounds. Include a variety in your daily diet.

**Choose Healthy Fats:**
Opt for sources of healthy fats, such as avocados, nuts, seeds, and olive oil. These fats have anti-inflammatory properties.

**Lean Proteins:**
Choose lean protein sources like fish, poultry, legumes, and tofu. These provide essential amino acids without excess saturated fat.

**Whole Grains:**
Replace refined grains with whole grains like quinoa, brown rice, and oats. These grains offer more fiber and nutrients.

**Hydration:**
Stay hydrated with water and herbal teas. Proper hydration supports overall health and may help control inflammation.

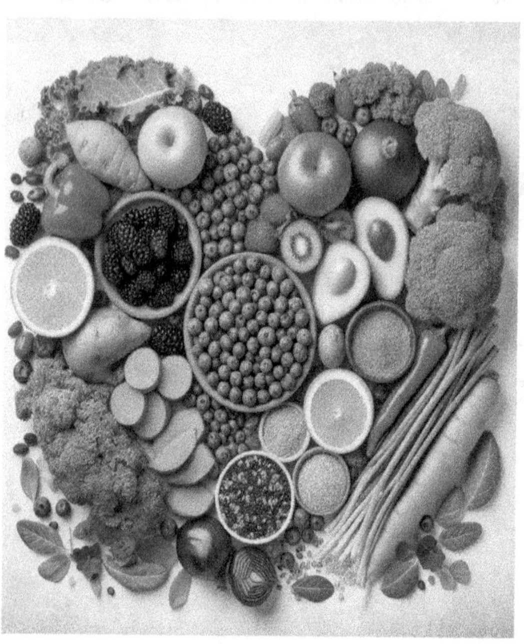

## Vegetables and vegetables products

**Broccoli:**
GI: Low
GL: Low
Sugar: 1.5g per 100g
Carbohydrates: 6g per 100g
Calories: 55 per 100g

**Spinach:**
GI: Low
GL: Low
Sugar: 0.4g per 100g
Carbohydrates: 3.6g per 100g
Calories: 23 per 100g

**Carrots:**
GI: Medium
GL: Low
Sugar: 4.7g per 100g
Carbohydrates: 10.7g per 100g
Calories: 41 per 100g

**Tomatoes:**
GI: Low
GL: Low
Sugar: 2.6g per 100g
Carbohydrates: 5.8g per 100g
Calories: 18 per 100g

**Bell Peppers:**
GI: Low
GL: Low
Sugar: 4.2g per 100g
Carbohydrates: 9.9g per 100g
Calories: 31 per 100g

**Cauliflower:**
GI: Low
GL: Low
Sugar: 1.9g per 100g
Carbohydrates: 5.3g per 100g
Calories: 25 per 100g

**Zucchini:**
GI: Low
GL: Low
Sugar: 2.1g per 100g
Carbohydrates: 3.1g per 100g
Calories: 17 per 100g

**Cabbage:**
GI: Low
GL: Low
Sugar: 2.2g per 100g
Carbohydrates: 5.8g per 100g
Calories: 25 per 100g

**Brussels Sprouts:**
GI: Low
GL: Low
Sugar: 2.2g per 100g
Carbohydrates: 8g per 100g
Calories: 43 per 100g

**Onions:**
GI: Low
GL: Low
Sugar: 4.7g per 100g
Carbohydrates: 9.3g per 100g
Calories: 40 per 100g

**Cucumber:**
GI: Low
GL: Low
Sugar: 1.7g per 100g
Carbohydrates: 3.6g per 100g
Calories: 15 per 100g

**Eggplant:**
GI: Low
GL: Low
Sugar: 3.5g per 100g
Carbohydrates: 8.6g per 100g
Calories: 25 per 100g

**Kale:**
GI: Low
GL: Low
Sugar: 0.9g per 100g
Carbohydrates: 8.8g per 100g
Calories: 49 per 100g

**Mushrooms:**
GI: Low
GL: Low
Sugar: 0.7g per 100g
Carbohydrates: 3.3g per 100g
Calories: 22 per 100g

**Artichokes:**
GI: Low
GL: Low
Sugar: 1g per 100g
Carbohydrates: 10.5g per 100g
Calories: 47 per 100g

**Turnips:**
GI: Low
GL: Low
Sugar: 4.4g per 100g
Carbohydrates: 8.4g per 100g
Calories: 28 per 100g

**Cilantro (Coriander):**
GI: Low
GL: Low
Sugar: 0.9g per 100g
Carbohydrates: 3.7g per 100g
Calories: 23 per 100g

**Radishes:**
GI: Low
GL: Low
Sugar: 1.9g per 100g
Carbohydrates: 3.4g per 100g
Calories: 16 per 100g

**Pumpkin:**
GI: Low
GL: Low
Sugar: 2.8g per 100g
Carbohydrates: 7g per 100g
Calories: 26 per 100g

**Squash (Butternut):**
GI: Low
GL: Low
Sugar: 2.2g per 100g
Carbohydrates: 11.7g per 100g
Calories: 45 per 100g

**Bell Peppers (Yellow):**
GI: Low
GL: Low
Sugar: 6g per 100g
Carbohydrates: 6g per 100g
Calories: 27 per 100g

**Lettuce (Romaine):**
GI: Low
GL: Low
Sugar: 1.2g per 100g
Carbohydrates: 3.3g per 100g
Calories: 17 per 100g

**Soybeans (Edamame):**
GI: Low
GL: Low
Sugar: 2.2g per 100g
Carbohydrates: 11.1g per 100g
Calories: 121 per 100g

**Bok Choy:**
GI: Low
GL: Low
Sugar: 1.2g per 100g
Carbohydrates: 2.2g per 100g
Calories: 13 per 100g

**Celery:**
GI: Low
GL: Low
Sugar: 1.8g per 100g
Carbohydrates: 3.8g per 100g
Calories: 16 per 100g

**Beets:**
GI: Medium
GL: Low
Sugar: 5.5g per 100g
Carbohydrates: 13g per 100g
Calories: 43 per 100g

**Garlic:**
GI: Low
GL: Low
Sugar: 1g per 100g
Carbohydrates: 33g per 100g
Calories: 149 per 100g

**Snap Peas:**
GI: Low
GL: Low
Sugar: 5.4g per 100g
Carbohydrates: 9g per 100g
Calories: 42 per 100g

**Fennel:**
GI: Low
GL: Low
Sugar: 3.9g per 100g
Carbohydrates: 7.3g per 100g
Calories: 31 per 100g

**Cabbage (Red):**
GI: Low
GL: Low
Sugar: 4.5g per 100g
Carbohydrates: 11.3g per 100g
Calories: 43 per 100g

**Berries Parfait:**

GI: Low

GL: Low

Sugar: 8g per cup

Carbohydrates: 25g per cup

Calories: 120 per cup


**Dark Chocolate-Covered Strawberries:**

GI: Low to medium

GL: Low

Sugar: 5g per 4 strawberries

Carbohydrates: 10g per 4 strawberries

Calories: 100 per 4 strawberries


**Chia Seed Pudding with Almond Milk:**

GI: Low

GL: Low

Sugar: 10g per 1/2 cup

Carbohydrates: 18g per 1/2 cup

Calories: 150 per 1/2 cup


**Yogurt Parfait with Nuts and Berries:**

GI: Low

GL: Low

Sugar: 12g per serving

Carbohydrates: 30g per serving

Calories: 200 per serving

**Baked Apples with Cinnamon:**
GI: Low
GL: Low
Sugar: 19g per apple
Carbohydrates: 25g per apple
Calories: 95 per apple

**Avocado Chocolate Mousse:**
GI: Low to medium
GL: Low
Sugar: 6g per 1/2 cup
Carbohydrates: 12g per 1/2 cup
Calories: 200 per 1/2 cup

**Coconut Flour Banana Bread:**
GI: Low
GL: Low
Sugar: 8g per slice
Carbohydrates: 20g per slice
Calories: 150 per slice

**Greek Yogurt Cheesecake:**
GI: Low
GL: Low
Sugar: 9g per slice
Carbohydrates: 15g per slice
Calories: 180 per slice

**Raspberry Almond Tart:**
GI: Low
GL: Low
Sugar: 12g per slice
Carbohydrates: 20g per slice
Calories: 220 per slice

**Pumpkin Chia Seed Pudding:**
GI: Low
GL: Low
Sugar: 8g per 1/2 cup
Carbohydrates: 15g per 1/2 cup
Calories: 130 per 1/2 cup

**Chocolate Avocado Ice Cream:**
GI: Low to medium
GL: Low
Sugar: 10g per 1/2 cup
Carbohydrates: 18g per 1/2 cup
Calories: 180 per 1/2 cup

**Almond Flour Lemon Poppy Seed Muffins:**
GI: Low
GL: Low
Sugar: 6g per muffin
Carbohydrates: 15g per muffin
Calories: 140 per muffin

**Strawberry Shortcake (with Coconut Flour):**
GI: Low
GL: Low
Sugar: 8g per serving
Carbohydrates: 18g per serving
Calories: 160 per serving

**Cocoa-Nut Energy Balls:**
GI: Low
GL: Low
Sugar: 5g per ball
Carbohydrates: 12g per ball
Calories: 120 per ball

**Peach and Almond Crumble:**
GI: Low
GL: Low
Sugar: 15g per serving
Carbohydrates: 30g per serving
Calories: 210 per serving

**Coconut Milk Rice Pudding:**
GI: Low
GL: Low
Sugar: 12g per 1/2 cup
Carbohydrates: 20g per 1/2 cup
Calories: 180 per 1/2 cup

**Blueberry Oat Bars:**

GI: Low

GL: Low

Sugar: 10g per bar

Carbohydrates: 25g per bar

Calories: 180 per bar

**Vanilla Bean Panna Cotta:**

GI: Low

GL: Low

Sugar: 8g per serving

Carbohydrates: 12g per serving

Calories: 150 per serving

**Cinnamon-Spiced Pears:**

GI: Low

GL: Low

Sugar: 18g per pear

Carbohydrates: 25g per pear

Calories: 100 per pear

**Mango Coconut Sorbet:**

GI: Low to medium

GL: Low

Sugar: 15g per 1/2 cup

Carbohydrates: 25g per 1/2 cup

Calories: 180 per 1/2 cup

**Chocolate Chia Seed Pudding:**
GI: Low
GL: Low
Sugar: 10g per 1/2 cup
Carbohydrates: 18g per 1/2 cup
Calories: 160 per 1/2 cup

**Almond Flour Chocolate Chip Cookies:**
GI: Low
GL: Low
Sugar: 5g per cookie
Carbohydrates: 12g per cookie
Calories: 120 per cookie

**Orange-Kissed Quinoa Pudding:**
GI: Low
GL: Low
Sugar: 10g per 1/2 cup
Carbohydrates: 20g per 1/2 cup
Calories: 160 per 1/2 cup

**Raspberry Almond Thumbprint Cookies:**
GI: Low
GL: Low
Sugar: 6g per cookie
Carbohydrates: 15g per cookie
Calories: 140 per cookie

**Apple Cinnamon Baked Oatmeal:**

GI: Low

GL: Low

Sugar: 10g per serving

Carbohydrates: 25g per serving

Calories: 180 per serving

**Coconut Flour Pumpkin Pie:**

GI: Low

GL: Low

Sugar: 15g per slice

Carbohydrates: 30g per slice

Calories: 220 per slice

**Pistachio and Cranberry Biscotti:**

GI: Low

GL: Low

Sugar: 8g per biscotti

Carbohydrates: 18g per biscotti

Calories: 160 per biscotti

**Vanilla Bean and Berry Custard:**

GI: Low

GL: Low

Sugar: 12g per serving

Carbohydrates: 20g per serving

Calories: 180 per serving

**Lemon Sorbet with Mint:**
GI: Low to medium
GL: Low
Sugar: 15g per 1/2 cup
Carbohydrates: 25g per 1/2 cup
Calories: 180 per 1/2 cup

**Chocolate Avocado Mousse Cake:**
GI: Low to medium
GL: Low
Sugar: 10g per slice
Carbohydrates: 25g per slice
Calories: 200 per slice

**Quinoa (GI: 53, GL: 13)**

Sugar: 0g

Carbohydrates: 30g per cup

Calories: 222 per cup


**Brown Rice Pasta (GI: 55, GL: 16)**

Sugar: 0g

Carbohydrates: 41g per cup

Calories: 218 per cup


**Gluten-Free Oats (GI: 55, GL: 13)**

Sugar: 1g

Carbohydrates: 28g per cup

Calories: 154 per cup

**Quinoa Flour (GI: 53, GL: 13)**

Sugar: 0g

Carbohydrates: 29g per cup

Calories: 120 per cup


**Chickpea Flour (GI: 44, GL: 9)**

Sugar: 1g

Carbohydrates: 22g per cup

Calories: 356 per cup


**Almond Flour (GI: 0, GL: 0)**

Sugar: 3g

Carbohydrates: 12g per cup

Calories: 580 per cup

**Coconut Flour (GI: 45, GL: 10)**

Sugar: 16g

Carbohydrates: 38g per cup

Calories: 480 per cup


**Buckwheat (GI: 54, GL: 10)**

Sugar: 1g

Carbohydrates: 34g per cup

Calories: 155 per cup


**Sweet Potato Noodles (GI: 44, GL: 11)**

Sugar: 7g

Carbohydrates: 41g per cup

Calories: 180 per cup

**Rice Flour (GI: 73, GL: 28) (use in moderation)**

Sugar: 0g

Carbohydrates: 120g per cup

Calories: 578 per cup


**Corn Flour (GI: 68, GL: 22) (use in moderation)**

Sugar: 0g

Carbohydrates: 115g per cup

Calories: 416 per cup


**Lentil Pasta (GI: 25, GL: 7)**

Sugar: 1g

Carbohydrates: 36g per cup

Calories: 210 per cup

**Tapioca Flour (GI: 68, GL: 23) (use in moderation)**

Sugar: 0g

Carbohydrates: 27g per cup

Calories: 544 per cup


**Sorghum Flour (GI: 66, GL: 22) (use in moderation)**

Sugar: 0g

Carbohydrates: 121g per cup

Calories: 620 per cup


**Millet (GI: 71, GL: 23) (use in moderation)**

Sugar: 1g

Carbohydrates: 174g per cup

Calories: 756 per cup

**Hazelnut Flour (GI: 0, GL: 0)**

Sugar: 2g

Carbohydrates: 16g per cup

Calories: 864 per cup


**Amaranth (GI: 65, GL: 23) (use in moderation)**

Sugar: 1g

Carbohydrates: 105g per cup

Calories: 716 per cup


**Arrowroot Flour (GI: 85, GL: 17) (use in moderation)**

Sugar: 0g

Carbohydrates: 111g per cup

Calories: 456 per cup

**Soy Flour (GI: 25, GL: 7)**

Sugar: 2g

Carbohydrates: 40g per cup

Calories: 424 per cup


**Chestnut Flour (GI: 54, GL: 9)**

Sugar: 11g

Carbohydrates: 103g per cup

Calories: 580 per cup


**Chia Seeds (GI: 1, GL: 0)**

Sugar: 0g

Carbohydrates: 12g per ounce

Calories: 138 per ounce

**Sunflower Seed Flour (GI: 30, GL: 7)**

Sugar: 0g

Carbohydrates: 18g per cup

Calories: 828 per cup


**Pumpkin Seed Flour (GI: 25, GL: 6)**

Sugar: 0g

Carbohydrates: 15g per cup

Calories: 504 per cup


**Cauliflower Rice (GI: 10, GL: 1)**

Sugar: 2g

Carbohydrates: 20g per cup

Calories: 27 per cup

**Brussels Sprouts (GI: 22, GL: 2)**

Sugar: 2g

Carbohydrates: 12g per cup

Calories: 38 per cup


**Eggplant (GI: 15, GL: 2)**

Sugar: 2g

Carbohydrates: 10g per cup

Calories: 20 per cup


**Cabbage (GI: 10, GL: 1)**

Sugar: 3g

Carbohydrates: 11g per cup

Calories: 22 per cup

**Green Beans (GI: 15, GL: 2)**

Sugar: 3g

Carbohydrates: 10g per cup

Calories: 31 per cup

**Mushrooms (GI: 10, GL: 1)**

Sugar: 1g

Carbohydrates: 5g per cup

Calories: 15 per cup

**Avocado (GI: 15, GL: 1)**

Sugar: 1g

Carbohydrates: 12g per cup

Calories: 240 per cup

**Amy's Organic Lentil Soup (Canned):**
GI: Low
GL: Low
Sugar: 1g per cup
Carbohydrates: 20g per cup
Calories: 180 per cup
Healthy Choice Simply Steamers Grilled Chicken and

**Broccoli Alfredo:**
GI: Low
GL: Low
Sugar: 3g per meal
Carbohydrates: 30g per meal
Calories: 300 per meal

**Caulipower Margherita Pizza (Frozen):**
GI: Low to medium
GL: Low
Sugar: 3g per serving
Carbohydrates: 36g per serving
Calories: 240 per serving

**Luvo Performance Kitchen Chicken Chile Verde:**
GI: Low
GL: Low
Sugar: 4g per bowl
Carbohydrates: 35g per bowl
Calories: 300 per bowl

**Evol Foods Butternut Squash and Sage Ravioli (Frozen):**
GI: Low to medium
GL: Low
Sugar: 6g per serving
Carbohydrates: 36g per serving
Calories: 290 per serving

**Kashi Chicken Florentine Frozen Bowl:**
GI: Low
GL: Low
Sugar: 2g per bowl
Carbohydrates: 34g per bowl
Calories: 260 per bowl

**Trader Joe's Quinoa Cowboy Veggie Burger (Frozen):**
GI: Low
GL: Low
Sugar: 1g per burger
Carbohydrates: 19g per burger
Calories: 160 per burger

**SmartMade Chicken with Spinach Fettuccine (Frozen):**
GI: Low
GL: Low
Sugar: 2g per meal
Carbohydrates: 27g per meal
Calories: 290 per meal

**Healthy Choice Power Bowls Cuban-Inspired Pork Bowl:**
GI: Low
GL: Low
Sugar: 5g per bowl
Carbohydrates: 36g per bowl
Calories: 330 per bowl

**Dr. Praeger's California Veggie Burger (Frozen):**
GI: Low
GL: Low
Sugar: 0g per burger
Carbohydrates: 9g per burger
Calories: 120 per burger

**Luvo Performance Kitchen Turkey Meatloaf and Mashed Potatoes:**
GI: Low
GL: Low
Sugar: 5g per bowl
Carbohydrates: 34g per bowl
Calories: 310 per bowl

**Cedarlane Quinoa and Vegetable Enchiladas (Frozen):**
GI: Low to medium
GL: Low
Sugar: 4g per serving
Carbohydrates: 39g per serving
Calories: 300 per serving

**Healthy Choice Simply Steamers Chicken and Vegetable Stir Fry:**
GI: Low
GL: Low
Sugar: 3g per meal
Carbohydrates: 27g per meal
Calories: 230 per meal

**EVOL Foods Fire Grilled Steak Bowl:**
GI: Low
GL: Low
Sugar: 2g per bowl
Carbohydrates: 29g per bowl
Calories: 270 per bowl

**Amy's Light & Lean Quinoa and Black Beans with Butternut Squash and Chard:**
GI: Low
GL: Low
Sugar: 4g per bowl
Carbohydrates: 32g per bowl
Calories: 240 per bowl

**Kashi 7 Whole Grain Pilaf (Frozen):**
GI: Low
GL: Low
Sugar: 1g per serving
Carbohydrates: 41g per serving
Calories: 180 per serving

**Lean Cuisine Features Butternut Squash Ravioli:**
GI: Low to medium
GL: Low
Sugar: 4g per meal
Carbohydrates: 35g per meal
Calories: 270 per meal

**Sweet Earth Enlightened Foods General Tso's Tofu (Frozen):**
GI: Low to medium
GL: Low
Sugar: 6g per serving
Carbohydrates: 41g per serving
Calories: 290 per serving

**Trader Joe's Shrimp Stir-Fry (Frozen):**
GI: Low
GL: Low
Sugar: 4g per serving
Carbohydrates: 27g per serving
Calories: 240 per serving

**EVOL Foods Truffle Parmesan Mac & Cheese (Frozen):**
GI: Low to medium
GL: Low
Sugar: 3g per bowl
Carbohydrates: 30g per bowl
Calories: 350 per bowl

**Cedarlane Eggplant Parmesan (Frozen):**
GI: Low to medium
GL: Low
Sugar: 5g per serving
Carbohydrates: 34g per serving
Calories: 310 per serving

**Healthy Choice Power Bowls Adobo Chicken Bowl:**
GI: Low
GL: Low
Sugar: 4g per bowl
Carbohydrates: 35g per bowl
Calories: 300 per bowl

**Dr. Praeger's Mushroom Risotto Veggie Burger (Frozen):**
GI: Low
GL: Low
Sugar: 1g per burger
Carbohydrates: 10g per burger
Calories: 140 per burger

**Luvo Performance Kitchen Chicken Harissa & Chickpeas:**
GI: Low
GL: Low
Sugar: 4g per bowl
Carbohydrates: 30g per bowl
Calories: 270 per bowl

**Amy's Pad Thai (Frozen):**

GI: Low to medium

GL: Low

Sugar: 4g per serving

Carbohydrates: 47g per serving

Calories: 320 per serving

**EVOL Foods Chicken Enchilada Bake:**

GI: Low

GL: Low

Sugar: 4g per bowl

Carbohydrates: 30g per bowl

Calories: 310 per bowl

**Healthy Choice Power Bowls Spicy Beef Teriyaki Bowl:**

GI: Low

GL: Low

Sugar: 4g per bowl

Carbohydrates: 36g per bowl

Calories: 330 per bowl

**Sweet Earth Enlightened Foods Kyoto Stir Fry (Frozen):**

GI: Low

GL: Low

Sugar: 5g per serving

Carbohydrates: 35g per serving

Calories: 300 per serving

**Caulipower Chicken Tenders (Frozen):**
GI: Low
GL: Low
Sugar: 0g per serving
Carbohydrates: 12g per serving
Calories: 490 per serving

**EVOL Foods Chicken Tikka Masala:**
GI: Low
GL: Low
Sugar: 3g per bowl
Carbohydrates: 31g per bowl
Calories: 310 per bowl

## Fruits and fruits products

**Apples:**
GI: Low to medium
GL: Low
Sugar: 10g per 100g
Carbohydrates: 14g per 100g
Calories: 52 per 100g

**Bananas:**
GI: Medium
GL: Medium
Sugar: 12g per 100g
Carbohydrates: 27g per 100g
Calories: 89 per 100g

**Berries (Mixed):**
GI: Low
GL: Low
Sugar: Varies (e.g., 5g for strawberries per 100g)
Carbohydrates: Varies
Calories: Varies

**Oranges:**
GI: Low
GL: Low
Sugar: 8.3g per 100g
Carbohydrates: 8.2g per 100g
Calories: 43 per 100g

**Grapes:**
GI: Medium
GL: Medium
Sugar: 16g per 100g
Carbohydrates: 18g per 100g
Calories: 69 per 100g

**Pineapple:**
GI: Medium
GL: Medium
Sugar: 9.9g per 100g
Carbohydrates: 13.1g per 100g
Calories: 50 per 100g

**Kiwi:**
GI: Low
GL: Low
Sugar: 9g per 100g
Carbohydrates: 14.6g per 100g
Calories: 61 per 100g

**Watermelon:**
GI: High
GL: Low
Sugar: 6.2g per 100g
Carbohydrates: 8.2g per 100g
Calories: 30 per 100g

**Peaches:**
GI: Low to medium
GL: Low
Sugar: 8.4g per 100g
Carbohydrates: 9.5g per 100g
Calories: 39 per 100g

**Mango:**
GI: Medium
GL: Medium
Sugar: 14.98g per 100g
Carbohydrates: 14.98g per 100g
Calories: 60 per 100g

**Plums:**
GI: Low to medium
GL: Low
Sugar: 9.92g per 100g
Carbohydrates: 11.42g per 100g
Calories: 46 per 100g

**Avocado:**
GI: Low
GL: Low
Sugar: 0.66g per 100g
Carbohydrates: 8.53g per 100g
Calories: 160 per 100g

**Cherries:**
GI: Low to medium
GL: Low
Sugar: 8.49g per 100g
Carbohydrates: 18.97g per 100g
Calories: 50 per 100g

**Pears:**
GI: Low to medium
GL: Low
Sugar: 9.8g per 100g
Carbohydrates: 14.29g per 100g
Calories: 57 per 100g

**Cranberries (fresh):**
GI: Low
GL: Low
Sugar: 4.04g per 100g
Carbohydrates: 12.2g per 100g
Calories: 46 per 100g

**Raspberries:**
GI: Low
GL: Low
Sugar: 4.42g per 100g
Carbohydrates: 11.94g per 100g
Calories: 52 per 100g

**Blueberries:**
GI: Low
GL: Low
Sugar: 9.68g per 100g
Carbohydrates: 14.49g per 100g
Calories: 57 per 100g

**Strawberries:**
GI: Low
GL: Low
Sugar: 4.89g per 100g
Carbohydrates: 7.68g per 100g
Calories: 32 per 100g

**Grapefruit:**
GI: Low
GL: Low
Sugar: 6.89g per 100g
Carbohydrates: 8.41g per 100g
Calories: 33 per 100g

**Apricots:**
GI: Low to medium
GL: Low
Sugar: 3.89g per 100g
Carbohydrates: 11.12g per 100g
Calories: 48 per 100g

**Dragon Fruit:**
GI: Low
GL: Low
Sugar: 8.06g per 100g
Carbohydrates: 9g per 100g
Calories: 60 per 100g

**Guava:**
GI: Low to medium
GL: Low
Sugar: 5.4g per 100g
Carbohydrates: 14g per 100g
Calories: 68 per 100g

**Passion Fruit:**
GI: Low
GL: Low
Sugar: 11.2g per 100g
Carbohydrates: 23.38g per 100g
Calories: 97 per 100g

**Cantaloupe:**
GI: Medium
GL: Low
Sugar: 8.2g per 100g
Carbohydrates: 8.16g per 100g
Calories: 34 per 100g

**Papaya:**
GI: Low
GL: Low
Sugar: 5.9g per 100g
Carbohydrates: 11g per 100g
Calories: 43 per 100g

**Kiwi (Gold):**
GI: Low
GL: Low
Sugar: 8.99g per 100g
Carbohydrates: 14.66g per 100g
Calories: 61 per 100g

**Blackberries:**
GI: Low
GL: Low
Sugar: 4.49g per 100g
Carbohydrates: 9.61g per 100g
Calories: 43 per 100g

**Currants (Black):**
GI: Low
GL: Low
Sugar: 7.37g per 100g
Carbohydrates: 18.4g per 100g
Calories: 63 per 100g

**Lychee:**
GI: Low to medium
GL: Low
Sugar: 9.2g per 100g
Carbohydrates: 21.6g per 100g
Calories: 66 per 100g

**Nectarines:**
GI: Low to medium
GL: Low
Sugar: 8.39g per 100g
Carbohydrates: 11.3g per 100g
Calories: 44 per 100g

**Turkey Sausage Links:**
Carbohydrates: 1g per link
Sugar: 0g
Calories: 50 per link

**Chicken Hot Dogs:**
Carbohydrates: 2g per hot dog
Sugar: 0g
Calories: 60 per hot dog

**Smoked Turkey Breast (Sliced):**
Carbohydrates: 0g per 2 slices
Sugar: 0g
Calories: 50 per 2 slices

**Beef Jerky (Low Sugar):**
Carbohydrates: 3g per ounce
Sugar: 2g
Calories: 70 per ounce

**Pork Bacon:**
Carbohydrates: 0g per slice
Sugar: 0g
Calories: 42 per slice

**Salami (Uncured):**
Carbohydrates: 0.5g per slice
Sugar: 0g
Calories: 60 per slice

**Chicken Breast Deli Slices:**
Carbohydrates: 1g per 3 slices
Sugar: 0g
Calories: 50 per 3 slices

**Turkey Pepperoni:**
Carbohydrates: 0g per 15 slices
Sugar: 0g
Calories: 70 per 15 slices

**Corned Beef (Canned):**
Carbohydrates: 0g per 2 ounces
Sugar: 0g
Calories: 90 per 2 ounces

**Pastrami (Sliced):**
Carbohydrates: 0.5g per slice
Sugar: 0g
Calories: 30 per slice

**Chicken Sausages (Spinach and Feta):**
Carbohydrates: 2g per link
Sugar: 0g
Calories: 80 per link

**Turkey Bacon:**
Carbohydrates: 0g per slice
Sugar: 0g
Calories: 35 per slice

**Roast Beef (Deli Style):**
Carbohydrates: 1g per 2 slices
Sugar: 0g
Calories: 60 per 2 slices

**Canadian Bacon**:
Carbohydrates: 1g per slice
Sugar: 0g
Calories: 30 per slice

**Turkey Ham:**
Carbohydrates: 1g per 2 ounces
Sugar: 0g
Calories: 50 per 2 ounces

**Chicken Salami:**
Carbohydrates: 0g per slice
Sugar: 0g
Calories: 30 per slice

**Pork Sausages (Uncured):**
Carbohydrates: 0g per link
Sugar: 0g
Calories: 80 per link

**Smoked Salmon (Sliced):**
Carbohydrates: 0g per 2 slices
Sugar: 0g
Calories: 60 per 2 slices

**Turkey Pastrami:**
Carbohydrates: 1g per 2 ounces
Sugar: 0g
Calories: 60 per 2 ounces

**Buffalo Chicken Wings (Grilled):**
Carbohydrates: 1g per wing
Sugar: 0g
Calories: 43 per wing

**Ham (Sliced):**
Carbohydrates: 1g per 2 slices
Sugar: 0g
Calories: 40 per 2 slices

**Turkey Burgers (Frozen):**
Carbohydrates: 0g per patty
Sugar: 0g
Calories: 150 per patty

**Peppered Turkey Jerky:**
Carbohydrates: 3g per ounce
Sugar: 2g
Calories: 80 per ounce

**Lamb Gyro Slices:**
Carbohydrates: 2g per 2 ounces
Sugar: 0g
Calories: 120 per 2 ounces

**Sliced Chicken Bologna:**
Carbohydrates: 1g per slice
Sugar: 0g
Calories: 40 per slice

**Grilled Chicken Strips (Pre-packaged):**
Carbohydrates: 0g per 3 ounces
Sugar: 0g
Calories: 90 per 3 ounces

**Prosciutto (Thinly Sliced):**
Carbohydrates: 0g per slice
Sugar: 0g
Calories: 30 per slice

**Tuna Salad (Pre-packaged):**
Carbohydrates: 4g per container
Sugar: 1g
Calories: 200 per container

**Chicken Teriyaki Sausages:**
Carbohydrates: 3g per link
Sugar: 0g
Calories: 70 per link

**Pulled Pork (Pre-packaged):**
Carbohydrates: 2g per 3 ounces
Sugar: 1g
Calories: 110 per 3 ounces

**Dark Chocolate (70% Cocoa):**
Carbohydrates: 14g per ounce
Sugar: 7g
Calories: 150 per ounce

**Sugar-Free Chocolate Bars:**
Carbohydrates: Varies by brand, typically 10g or less per serving
Sugar: Varies by brand, typically 0g per serving
Calories: Varies by brand, typically 100 calories or less per serving

**Dark Chocolate-Covered Almonds:**
Carbohydrates: 18g per 1/4 cup
Sugar: 8g
Calories: 210 per 1/4 cup

**Stevia-Sweetened Chocolate:**
Carbohydrates: Varies by brand, typically 10g or less per serving
Sugar: Varies by brand, typically 0g per serving
Calories: Varies by brand, typically 100 calories or less per serving

**Sugar-Free Gummy Bears:**
Carbohydrates: Varies by brand, typically 10g or less per serving
Sugar: Varies by brand, typically 0g per serving
Calories: Varies by brand, typically 100 calories or less per serving

**Dark Chocolate-Covered Strawberries:**
Carbohydrates: 15g per 1/4 cup
Sugar: 10g
Calories: 180 per 1/4 cup

**Sugar-Free Hard Candy (Various Flavors):**
Carbohydrates: Varies by brand, typically 5g or less per serving
Sugar: Varies by brand, typically 0g per serving
Calories: Varies by brand, typically 30 calories or less per serving

**Cocoa-Dusted Almonds:**
Carbohydrates: 18g per 1/4 cup
Sugar: 8g
Calories: 210 per 1/4 cup

**Dark Chocolate-Covered Blueberries:**
Carbohydrates: 15g per 1/4 cup
Sugar: 10g
Calories: 180 per 1/4 cup

**Coconut-Flour Chocolate Brownies:**
Carbohydrates: Varies by recipe, typically 15g or less per serving
Sugar: Varies by recipe, typically 5g or less per serving
Calories: Varies by recipe, typically 150 calories or less per serving

**Sugar-Free Licorice:**
Carbohydrates: Varies by brand, typically 10g or less per serving
Sugar: Varies by brand, typically 0g per serving
Calories: Varies by brand, typically 100 calories or less per serving

**Dark Chocolate-Covered Raspberries:**
Carbohydrates: 15g per 1/4 cup
Sugar: 10g
Calories: 180 per 1/4 cup

**Stevia-Sweetened Gumdrops:**
Carbohydrates: Varies by brand, typically 10g or less per serving
Sugar: Varies by brand, typically 0g per serving
Calories: Varies by brand, typically 100 calories or less per serving

**Dark Chocolate-Covered Cranberries:**
Carbohydrates: 15g per 1/4 cup
Sugar: 10g
Calories: 180 per 1/4 cup

**Sugar-Free Caramel Chews:**
Carbohydrates: Varies by brand, typically 10g or less per serving
Sugar: Varies by brand, typically 0g per serving
Calories: Varies by brand, typically 100 calories or less per serving

**Cacao Nibs:**
Carbohydrates: 12g per ounce
Sugar: 0g
Calories: 130 per ounce

**Dark Chocolate-Covered Cherries:**
Carbohydrates: 15g per 1/4 cup
Sugar: 10g
Calories: 180 per 1/4 cup

**Sugar-Free Peanut Butter Cups:**
Carbohydrates: Varies by brand, typically 10g or less per serving
Sugar: Varies by brand, typically 0g per serving
Calories: Varies by brand, typically 100 calories or less per serving

**Dark Chocolate-Covered Hazelnuts:**
Carbohydrates: 18g per 1/4 cup
Sugar: 8g
Calories: 210 per 1/4 cup

**Stevia-Sweetened Chocolate Chips:**
Carbohydrates: Varies by brand, typically 10g or less per 1/4 cup
Sugar: Varies by brand, typically 0g per 1/4 cup
Calories: Varies by brand, typically 100 calories or less per 1/4 cup

**Sugar-Free Toffee:**
Carbohydrates: Varies by brand, typically 10g or less per serving
Sugar: Varies by brand, typically 0g per serving
Calories: Varies by brand, typically 100 calories or less per serving

***Dark Chocolate-Covered Apricots:***
Carbohydrates: 15g per 1/4 cup
Sugar: 10g
Calories: 180 per 1/4 cup

**Sugar-Free Jelly Beans:**
Carbohydrates: Varies by brand, typically 10g or less per serving
Sugar: Varies by brand, typically 0g per serving
Calories: Varies by brand, typically 100 calories or less per serving

***Dark Chocolate-Covered Pineapple:***
Carbohydrates: 15g per 1/4 cup
Sugar: 10g
Calories: 180 per 1/4 cup

**Stevia-Sweetened Caramel Sauce:**
Carbohydrates: Varies by brand, typically 10g or less per serving
Sugar: Varies by brand, typically 0g per serving
Calories: Varies by brand, typically 100 calories or less per serving

***Dark Chocolate-Covered Mango:***
Carbohydrates: 15g per 1/4 cup
Sugar: 10g
Calories: 180 per 1/4 cup

**Sugar-Free Marshmallows:**
Carbohydrates: Varies by brand, typically 10g or less per serving
Sugar: Varies by brand, typically 0g per serving
Calories: Varies by brand, typically 100 calories or less per serving

**Dark Chocolate-Covered Goji Berries:**
Carbohydrates: 15g per 1/4 cup
Sugar: 10g
Calories: 180 per 1/4 cup

**Sugar-Free Peppermint Patties:**
Carbohydrates: Varies by brand, typically 10g or less per serving
Sugar: Varies by brand, typically 0g per serving
Calories: Varies by brand, typically 100 calories or less per serving

**Dark Chocolate-Covered Pistachios:**
Carbohydrates: 18g per 1/4 cup
Sugar: 8g
Calories: 210 per 1/4 cup

## Vegetarians and vegan foods

**Lentils (Cooked):**
GI: Low
GL: Low
Sugar: 0.8g per cup
Carbohydrates: 39.9g per cup
Calories: 230 per cup

**Chickpeas (Cooked):**
GI: Low
GL: Low
Sugar: 4.7g per cup
Carbohydrates: 45g per cup
Calories: 269 per cup

**Quinoa (Cooked):**
GI: Low
GL: Low
Sugar: 0.9g per cup
Carbohydrates: 39.4g per cup
Calories: 222 per cup

**Black Beans (Cooked):**
GI: Low
GL: Low
Sugar: 0.5g per cup
Carbohydrates: 40.8g per cup
Calories: 227 per cup

**Edamame (Cooked):**
GI: Low
GL: Low
Sugar: 3.7g per cup
Carbohydrates: 15.4g per cup
Calories: 189 per cup

**Tempeh:**
GI: Low
GL: Low
Sugar: 0.6g per 3-ounce serving
Carbohydrates: 7g per 3-ounce serving
Calories: 160 per 3-ounce serving

**Tofu:**
GI: Low
GL: Low
Sugar: 0.1g per 3-ounce serving
Carbohydrates: 1.9g per 3-ounce serving
Calories: 70 per 3-ounce serving

**Brown Rice (Cooked):**
GI: Low to medium
GL: Low
Sugar: 0.2g per cup
Carbohydrates: 45.8g per cup
Calories: 215 per cup

**Spinach (Raw):**
GI: Low
GL: Low
Sugar: 0.1g per cup
Carbohydrates: 6.7g per cup
Calories: 7 per cup

**Cauliflower (Raw):**
GI: Low
GL: Low
Sugar: 2.5g per cup
Carbohydrates: 5.3g per cup
Calories: 27 per cup

**Almonds:**
GI: Low
GL: Low
Sugar: 0.7g per ounce
Carbohydrates: 5.6g per ounce
Calories: 160 per ounce

**Avocado**:
GI: Low
GL: Low
Sugar: 0.2g per ounce
Carbohydrates: 8.5g per ounce
Calories: 50 per ounce

**Zucchini (Raw):**
GI: Low
GL: Low
Sugar: 2.2g per cup
Carbohydrates: 3.9g per cup
Calories: 20 per cup

**Broccoli (Raw):**
GI: Low
GL: Low
Sugar: 1.5g per cup
Carbohydrates: 6g per cup
Calories: 31 per cup

**Sweet Potatoes (Baked):**
GI: Medium
GL: Low to medium
Sugar: 7.4g per medium potato
Carbohydrates: 26.8g per medium potato
Calories: 103 per medium potato

**Kale (Raw):**
GI: Low
GL: Low
Sugar: 0.6g per cup
Carbohydrates: 6g per cup
Calories: 33 per cup

**Brussels Sprouts (Raw):**
GI: Low
GL: Low
Sugar: 1.9g per cup
Carbohydrates: 8g per cup
Calories: 38 per cup

**Artichokes (Steamed):**
GI: Low
GL: Low
Sugar: 1g per artichoke
Carbohydrates: 13.4g per artichoke
Calories: 60 per artichoke

**Mushrooms (Raw):**
GI: Low
GL: Low
Sugar: 1g per cup
Carbohydrates: 2.3g per cup
Calories: 15 per cup

**Pumpkin (Baked):**
GI: Low
GL: Low
Sugar: 1.2g per cup
Carbohydrates: 12.8g per cup
Calories: 49 per cup

**Cabbage (Raw):**
GI: Low
GL: Low
Sugar: 2.2g per cup
Carbohydrates: 5.8g per cup
Calories: 22 per cup

**Cucumber (Raw):**
GI: Low
GL: Low
Sugar: 1.9g per cup
Carbohydrates: 3.8g per cup
Calories: 16 per cup

**Bell Peppers (Raw):**
GI: Low
GL: Low
Sugar: 3.9g per cup
Carbohydrates: 9.9g per cup
Calories: 46 per cup

**Chia Seeds:**
GI: Low
GL: Low
Sugar: 0g per ounce
Carbohydrates: 12g per ounce
Calories: 138 per ounce

**Sunflower Seeds:**
GI: Low
GL: Low
Sugar: 0.7g per ounce
Carbohydrates: 6.9g per ounce
Calories: 161 per ounce

**Cilantro (Raw):**
GI: Low
GL: Low
Sugar: 0.1g per cup
Carbohydrates: 0.3g per cup
Calories: 0 per cup

**Ginger (Raw):**
GI: Low
GL: Low
Sugar: 0.6g per tablespoon
Carbohydrates: 1.7g per tablespoon
Calories: 5 per tablespoon

**Asparagus (Raw):**
GI: Low
GL: Low
Sugar: 0.6g per spear
Carbohydrates: 1.3g per spear
Calories: 3 per spear

**Celery (Raw):**
GI: Low
GL: Low
Sugar: 0.8g per cup
Carbohydrates: 1.9g per cup
Calories: 16 per cup

**Eggplant (Grilled):**
GI: Low
GL: Low
Sugar: 2.5g per cup
Carbohydrates: 10.4g per cup
Calories: 20 per cup

**Whole Grain Bread:**

GI: Low

GL: Low

Sugar: 2g per slice

Carbohydrates: 15g per slice

Calories: 80 per slice

**Ezekiel Bread:**

GI: Low

GL: Low

Sugar: 0g per slice

Carbohydrates: 15g per slice

Calories: 80 per slice

**Oat Bran Muffins:**

GI: Low to medium

GL: Low

Sugar: 5g per muffin

Carbohydrates: 25g per muffin

Calories: 120 per muffin

**Barley Bread:**

GI: Low

GL: Low

Sugar: 1g per slice

Carbohydrates: 15g per slice

Calories: 70 per slice

**Sourdough Bread:**
GI: Low
GL: Low
Sugar: 1g per slice
Carbohydrates: 15g per slice
Calories: 80 per slice

**Multigrain Bagel:**
GI: Low to medium
GL: Low
Sugar: 3g per bagel
Carbohydrates: 45g per bagel
Calories: 240 per bagel

**Whole Wheat English Muffin:**
GI: Low
GL: Low
Sugar: 1g per muffin
Carbohydrates: 24g per muffin
Calories: 130 per muffin

**Spelt Bread:**
GI: Low
GL: Low
Sugar: 1g per slice
Carbohydrates: 15g per slice
Calories: 70 per slice

**Brown Rice Flour Pancakes:**

GI: Low

GL: Low

Sugar: 2g per pancake

Carbohydrates: 20g per pancake

Calories: 100 per pancake

**Chia Seed Muffins:**

GI: Low to medium

GL: Low

Sugar: 3g per muffin

Carbohydrates: 25g per muffin

Calories: 120 per muffin

**Almond Flour Bread:**

GI: Low

GL: Low

Sugar: 1g per slice

Carbohydrates: 3g per slice

Calories: 50 per slice

**Buckwheat Pancakes:**

GI: Low

GL: Low

Sugar: 2g per pancake

Carbohydrates: 20g per pancake

Calories: 100 per pancake

**Quinoa Bread:**
GI: Low
GL: Low
Sugar: 2g per slice
Carbohydrates: 15g per slice
Calories: 80 per slice

**Rye Bread:**
GI: Low
GL: Low
Sugar: 1g per slice
Carbohydrates: 15g per slice
Calories: 80 per slice

**Coconut Flour Muffins:**
GI: Low to medium
GL: Low
Sugar: 4g per muffin
Carbohydrates: 15g per muffin
Calories: 120 per muffin

**Sweet Potato Scones**:
GI: Low to medium
GL: Low
Sugar: 5g per scone
Carbohydrates: 30g per scone
Calories: 150 per scone

**Chickpea Flour Flatbread (Socca):**
GI: Low
GL: Low
Sugar: 2g per slice
Carbohydrates: 15g per slice
Calories: 80 per slice

**Whole Wheat Pita Bread:**
GI: Low
GL: Low
Sugar: 2g per pita
Carbohydrates: 33g per pita
Calories: 170 per pita

**Hazelnut Flour Muffins:**
GI: Low to medium
GL: Low
Sugar: 4g per muffin
Carbohydrates: 15g per muffin
Calories: 120 per muffin

**Amaranth Bread:**
GI: Low
GL: Low
Sugar: 1g per slice
Carbohydrates: 15g per slice
Calories: 80 per slice

**Pumpernickel Bread:**
GI: Low
GL: Low
Sugar: 1g per slice
Carbohydrates: 15g per slice
Calories: 80 per slice

**Cinnamon Raisin Bread (Whole Grain):**
GI: Low to medium
GL: Low
Sugar: 5g per slice
Carbohydrates: 30g per slice
Calories: 140 per slice

**Sunflower Seed Bread:**
GI: Low
GL: Low
Sugar: 1g per slice
Carbohydrates: 15g per slice
Calories: 80 per slice

**Whole Wheat Tortillas:**
GI: Low
GL: Low
Sugar: 2g per tortilla
Carbohydrates: 24g per tortilla
Calories: 120 per tortilla

**Sesame Seed Bread:**

GI: Low
GL: Low
Sugar: 1g per slice
Carbohydrates: 15g per slice
Calories: 80 per slice

**Pear and Walnut Muffins:**

GI: Low to medium
GL: Low
Sugar: 6g per muffin
Carbohydrates: 30g per muffin
Calories: 150 per muffin

**Rye Crispbread:**

GI: Low
GL: Low
Sugar: 0.5g per crispbread
Carbohydrates: 15g per 4 crispbreads
Calories: 70 per 4 crispbreads

**Hazelnut Cranberry Biscuits:**

GI: Low to medium
GL: Low
Sugar: 7g per biscuit
Carbohydrates: 25g per biscuit
Calories: 130 per biscuit

**Walnut Banana Bread:**
GI: Low to medium
GL: Low
Sugar: 8g per slice
Carbohydrates: 30g per slice
Calories: 150 per slice

**Flaxseed Bread:**
GI: Low
GL: Low
Sugar: 1g per slice
Carbohydrates: 15g per slice
Calories: 80 per slice

## Eggs

**Whole Eggs (Boiled):**
GI: Low
GL: Low
Sugar: 0.6g per large egg
Carbohydrates: 0.6g per large egg
Calories: 68 per large egg

**Egg Whites (Cooked):**
GI: Low
GL: Low
Sugar: 0g per cup
Carbohydrates: 0.6g per cup
Calories: 126 per cup

**Scrambled Eggs (Cooked with Milk):**
GI: Low
GL: Low
Sugar: 1.4g per cup
Carbohydrates: 3.6g per cup
Calories: 251 per cup

**Hard-Boiled Egg Whites:**
GI: Low
GL: Low
Sugar: 0g per egg white
Carbohydrates: 0.2g per egg white
Calories: 17 per egg white

**Omelette (with Vegetables):**
GI: Low
GL: Low
Sugar: 1.8g per omelette
Carbohydrates: 3.4g per omelette
Calories: 94 per omelette

**Poached Eggs:**
GI: Low
GL: Low
Sugar: 0.6g per egg
Carbohydrates: 0.6g per egg
Calories: 68 per egg

**Boiled Eggs (Deviled):**
GI: Low
GL: Low
Sugar: 0.4g per half egg
Carbohydrates: 0.1g per half egg
Calories: 63 per half egg

**Fried Eggs (Cooked in Olive Oil):**
GI: Low
GL: Low
Sugar: 0g per egg
Carbohydrates: 0.6g per egg
Calories: 90 per egg

**Egg Salad (Homemade):**
GI: Low
GL: Low
Sugar: 0.9g per cup
Carbohydrates: 2.1g per cup
Calories: 220 per cup

**Egg Drop Soup:**
GI: Low
GL: Low
Sugar: 0.5g per cup
Carbohydrates: 1.3g per cup
Calories: 68 per cup

**Quiche (Crustless):**
GI: Low
GL: Low
Sugar: 1.3g per slice
Carbohydrates: 3.1g per slice
Calories: 99 per slice

**Egg Muffins (with Spinach and Feta):**
GI: Low
GL: Low
Sugar: 0.5g per muffin
Carbohydrates: 1.9g per muffin
Calories: 71 per muffin

**Egg Curry:**
GI: Low
GL: Low
Sugar: 0.6g per serving
Carbohydrates: 1.2g per serving
Calories: 94 per serving

**Egg and Avocado Wrap:**
GI: Low
GL: Low
Sugar: 1g per wrap
Carbohydrates: 4.5g per wrap
Calories: 201 per wrap

**Shakshuka (Poached Eggs in Tomato Sauce):**
GI: Low
GL: Low
Sugar: 4g per serving
Carbohydrates: 10g per serving
Calories: 160 per serving

**Egg Casserole (with Vegetables):**
GI: Low
GL: Low
Sugar: 1.2g per serving
Carbohydrates: 2.4g per serving
Calories: 115 per serving

**Egg Fried Rice (with Cauliflower Rice):**
GI: Low
GL: Low
Sugar: 1.5g per cup
Carbohydrates: 6.2g per cup
Calories: 150 per cup

**Egg and Cheese Stuffed Bell Peppers:**
GI: Low
GL: Low
Sugar: 1.3g per serving
Carbohydrates: 4.7g per serving
Calories: 93 per serving

**Egg and Tomato Breakfast Sandwich:**
GI: Low
GL: Low
Sugar: 2.4g per sandwich
Carbohydrates: 24.6g per sandwich
Calories: 265 per sandwich

**Egg and Vegetable Stir-Fry:**
GI: Low
GL: Low
Sugar: 1.8g per serving
Carbohydrates: 5.7g per serving
Calories: 115 per serving

**Egg and Spinach Breakfast Burrito:**
GI: Low
GL: Low
Sugar: 1.5g per burrito
Carbohydrates: 27g per burrito
Calories: 200 per burrito

**Egg and Mushroom Skewers:**
GI: Low
GL: Low
Sugar: 0.8g per skewer
Carbohydrates: 2g per skewer
Calories: 40 per skewer

**Egg Noodle Stir-Fry (with Zucchini Noodles):**
GI: Low
GL: Low
Sugar: 2g per cup
Carbohydrates: 8g per cup
Calories: 55 per cup

**Egg and Cauliflower Bites:**
GI: Low
GL: Low
Sugar: 0.9g per bite
Carbohydrates: 1.9g per bite
Calories: 23 per bite

**Egg and Cabbage Skillet:**
GI: Low
GL: Low
Sugar: 2.3g per serving
Carbohydrates: 6.7g per serving
Calories: 102 per serving

*Egg and Salsa Wrap:*
GI: Low
GL: Low
Sugar: 1.7g per wrap
Carbohydrates: 20.3g per wrap
Calories: 240 per wrap

**Egg Stuffed Portobello Mushrooms:**
GI: Low
GL: Low
Sugar: 1.2g per mushroom
Carbohydrates: 3.4g per mushroom
Calories: 52 per mushroom

**Egg and Kale Breakfast Bowl:**
GI: Low
GL: Low
Sugar: 1.4g per bowl
Carbohydrates: 10.2g per bowl
Calories: 140 per bowl

**Egg and Cheese Quesadilla (with Whole Wheat Tortilla):**
GI: Low to medium
GL: Low
Sugar: 1.5g per quesadilla
Carbohydrates: 20g per quesadilla
Calories: 242 per quesadilla

**Egg and Broccoli Frittata:**
GI: Low
GL: Low
Sugar: 1.8g per serving
Carbohydrates: 4.5g per serving
Calories: 80 per serving

**Chicken Breast (Grilled):**
Carbohydrates: 0g
Protein: 31g per 100g
Fat: 3.6g per 100g
Calories: 165 per 100g

**Salmon (Baked):**
Carbohydrates: 0g
Protein: 25g per 100g
Fat: 10.5g per 100g
Calories: 206 per 100g

**Lean Ground Turkey (Cooked):**
Carbohydrates: 0g
Protein: 21g per 100g
Fat: 7.3g per 100g
Calories: 135 per 100g

**Tuna (Canned in Water):**
Carbohydrates: 0g
Protein: 29g per 100g
Fat: 1g per 100g
Calories: 132 per 100g

**Beef Tenderloin (Grilled):**
Carbohydrates: 0g
Protein: 36g per 100g
Fat: 8.6g per 100g
Calories: 250 per 100g

**Shrimp (Boiled):**
Carbohydrates: 0g
Protein: 24g per 100g
Fat: 1.5g per 100g
Calories: 99 per 100g

**Pork Chop (Grilled):**
Carbohydrates: 0g
Protein: 31g per 100g
Fat: 9g per 100g
Calories: 214 per 100g

**Cod (Baked):**
Carbohydrates: 0g
Protein: 20g per 100g
Fat: 1g per 100g
Calories: 105 per 100g

**Chicken Thigh (Roasted, Skinless):**
Carbohydrates: 0g
Protein: 26g per 100g
Fat: 10.5g per 100g
Calories: 187 per 100g

**Turkey Breast (Roasted, Skinless):**
Carbohydrates: 0g
Protein: 29g per 100g
Fat: 1g per 100g
Calories: 135 per 100g

**Lamb Chops (Grilled):**
Carbohydrates: 0g
Protein: 25g per 100g
Fat: 20g per 100g
Calories: 277 per 100g

**Scallops (Pan-Seared):**
Carbohydrates: 3.7g per 100g
Protein: 20g per 100g
Fat: 1.3g per 100g
Calories: 95 per 100g

**Lean Ground Beef (Cooked):**
Carbohydrates: 0g
Protein: 26g per 100g
Fat: 10g per 100g
Calories: 207 per 100g

*Sardines (Canned in Olive Oil):*
Carbohydrates: 0g
Protein: 21g per 100g
Fat: 11g per 100g
Calories: 208 per 100g

**Chicken Drumstick (Roasted, Skinless):**
Carbohydrates: 0g
Protein: 28g per 100g
Fat: 8.2g per 100g
Calories: 184 per 100g

**Halibut (Grilled):**
Carbohydrates: 0g
Protein: 21g per 100g
Fat: 2.3g per 100g
Calories: 119 per 100g

**Venison (Roasted):**
Carbohydrates: 0g
Protein: 30g per 100g
Fat: 4g per 100g
Calories: 158 per 100g

**Catfish (Baked):**
Carbohydrates: 0g
Protein: 22g per 100g
Fat: 7.4g per 100g
Calories: 148 per 100g

**Chicken Wings (Baked, Skinless):**
Carbohydrates: 0g
Protein: 30g per 100g
Fat: 8.6g per 100g
Calories: 203 per 100g

**Anchovies (Canned in Oil):**
Carbohydrates: 0g
Protein: 29g per 100g
Fat: 19g per 100g
Calories: 298 per 100g

**Turkey Leg (Roasted, Skinless):**
Carbohydrates: 0g
Protein: 28g per 100g
Fat: 3.6g per 100g
Calories: 155 per 100g

**Rainbow Trout (Baked):**
Carbohydrates: 0g
Protein: 22g per 100g
Fat: 9g per 100g
Calories: 169 per 100g

**Quail (Roasted):**
Carbohydrates: 0g
Protein: 25g per 100g
Fat: 7g per 100g
Calories: 158 per 100g

**Crab (Steamed):**
Carbohydrates: 0g
Protein: 18g per 100g
Fat: 1.1g per 100g
Calories: 84 per 100g

**Chicken Liver (Pan-Fried):**
Carbohydrates: 2.1g per 100g
Protein: 17g per 100g
Fat: 7.4g per 100g
Calories: 135 per 100g

**Mackerel (Grilled):**
Carbohydrates: 0g
Protein: 18g per 100g
Fat: 13g per 100g
Calories: 230 per 100g

**Duck Breast (Roasted, Skinless):**
Carbohydrates: 0g
Protein: 24g per 100g
Fat: 6g per 100g
Calories: 165 per 100g

**Tilapia (Baked):**
Carbohydrates: 0g
Protein: 21g per 100g
Fat: 1.7g per 100g
Calories: 96 per 100g

**Oysters (Raw):**
Carbohydrates: 4.3g per 100g
Protein: 9.8g per 100g
Fat: 2g per 100g
Calories: 68 per 100g

**Veal (Roasted):**
Carbohydrates: 0g
Protein: 30g per 100g
Fat: 7g per 100g
Calories: 189 per 100g

**Water:**
Carbohydrates: 0g
Sugar: 0g
Calories: 0

**Herbal Tea (Unsweetened):**
Carbohydrates: 0g
Sugar: 0g
Calories: 0

**Green Tea (Unsweetened):**
Carbohydrates: 0g
Sugar: 0g
Calories: 0

**Black Coffee (Unsweetened):**
Carbohydrates: 0g
Sugar: 0g
Calories: 2 (per 8 oz cup)

**Chamomile Tea (Unsweetened):**
Carbohydrates: 0g
Sugar: 0g
Calories: 0

**Sparkling Water (Unsweetened):**
Carbohydrates: 0g
Sugar: 0g
Calories: 0

**Ginger Tea (Unsweetened):**
Carbohydrates: 0g
Sugar: 0g
Calories: 0

**Peppermint Tea (Unsweetened):**
Carbohydrates: 0g
Sugar: 0g
Calories: 0

**Hibiscus Tea (Unsweetened):**
Carbohydrates: 0g
Sugar: 0g
Calories: 0

**Coconut Water (Natural, No Added Sugar):**
Carbohydrates: 9g per 100ml
Sugar: 5.5g per 100ml
Calories: 19 per 100ml

**Almond Milk (Unsweetened):**
Carbohydrates: 1g per cup
Sugar: 0g
Calories: 30 per cup

**Lemon Water (No Added Sugar):**
Carbohydrates: 2g per 8 oz
Sugar: 0.3g per 8 oz
Calories: 7 per 8 oz

**Iced Green Tea (Unsweetened):**
Carbohydrates: 0g
Sugar: 0g
Calories: 0

**Vegetable Juice (Low-Sodium):**
Carbohydrates: 9g per cup
Sugar: 5g per cup
Calories: 50 per cup

**Tomato Juice (Low-Sodium):**
Carbohydrates: 10g per cup
Sugar: 5g per cup
Calories: 50 per cup

**Black Tea (Unsweetened):**
Carbohydrates: 0g
Sugar: 0g
Calories: 2 (per 8 oz cup)

**Cranberry Juice (No Sugar Added):**
Carbohydrates: 10g per cup
Sugar: 4g per cup
Calories: 46 per cup

**Soy Milk (Unsweetened):**
Carbohydrates: 1g per cup
Sugar: 0g
Calories: 80 per cup

**Rooibos Tea (Unsweetened):**
Carbohydrates: 0g
Sugar: 0g
Calories: 0

**Kombucha (Unsweetened):**
Carbohydrates: 2-3g per cup
Sugar: Varies
Calories: Varies

**Wheatgrass Juice:**
Carbohydrates: 15g per 2 oz
Sugar: 0g
Calories: 80 per 2 oz

**Mint Tea (Unsweetened):**
Carbohydrates: 0g
Sugar: 0g
Calories: 0

**Chia Seed Drink (No Added Sugar):**
Carbohydrates: 15g per cup
Sugar: 0g
Calories: 60 per cup

**Oolong Tea (Unsweetened):**
Carbohydrates: 0g
Sugar: 0g
Calories: 2 (per 8 oz cup)

**Unsweetened Apple Cider Vinegar Drink:**
Carbohydrates: 0.1g per tablespoon
Sugar: 0g
Calories: 1 per tablespoon

**Hemp Milk (Unsweetened):**
Carbohydrates: 1g per cup
Sugar: 0g
Calories: 70 per cup

**Nettle Tea (Unsweetened):**
Carbohydrates: 0g
Sugar: 0g
Calories: 0

**Matcha Latte (Unsweetened, with Unsweetened Almond Milk):**
Carbohydrates: 1g per cup
Sugar: 0g
Calories: 30 per cup

**Cucumber Infused Water (No Added Sugar):**
Carbohydrates: 2g per cup
Sugar: 1g per cup
Calories: 8 per cup

**Rosehip Tea (Unsweetened):**
Carbohydrates: 0g
Sugar: 0g
Calories: 0

**Steel-Cut Oats:**
GI: Low
GL: Low
Sugar: 0g (unsweetened)
Carbohydrates: 27g per 100g (cooked)
Calories: 68 per 100g (cooked)

**Quinoa Flakes:**
GI: Low to medium
GL: Low
Sugar: 0g (unsweetened)
Carbohydrates: 21g per 100g (cooked)
Calories: 120 per 100g (cooked)

**Bran Flakes:**
GI: Medium
GL: Low
Sugar: 5g per 100g
Carbohydrates: 58g per 100g
Calories: 255 per 100g

**Muesli (No Added Sugar):**
GI: Low to medium
GL: Low
Sugar: 5g per 100g
Carbohydrates: 68g per 100g
Calories: 370 per 100g

**Shredded Wheat:**
GI: Low to medium
GL: Low
Sugar: 0g
Carbohydrates: 44g per 100g
Calories: 151 per 100g

**Oat Bran Cereal:**
GI: Low to medium
GL: Low
Sugar: 1g per 100g
Carbohydrates: 59g per 100g
Calories: 246 per 100g

**Barley Flakes:**
GI: Low to medium
GL: Low
Sugar: 0g (unsweetened)
Carbohydrates: 25g per 100g (cooked)
Calories: 123 per 100g (cooked)

**Brown Rice Cakes (Unsalted):**
GI: Low to medium
GL: Low
Sugar: 0g
Carbohydrates: 19g per 100g
Calories: 387 per 100g

**Buckwheat Groats (Kasha):**
GI: Low
GL: Low
Sugar: 1g per 100g (cooked)
Carbohydrates: 19g per 100g (cooked)
Calories: 92 per 100g (cooked)

**Wheat Bran:**
GI: Low
GL: Low
Sugar: 0g (unsweetened)
Carbohydrates: 39g per 100g
Calories: 125 per 100g

**Whole Grain Puffed Rice:**
GI: Low to medium
GL: Low
Sugar: 0g (unsweetened)
Carbohydrates: 80g per 100g
Calories: 402 per 100g

**Amaranth Flakes:**
GI: Low to medium
GL: Low
Sugar: 1g per 100g (cooked)
Carbohydrates: 19g per 100g (cooked)
Calories: 102 per 100g (cooked)

**Almond Flour Cereal:**
GI: Low
GL: Low
Sugar: 2g per 100g
Carbohydrates: 22g per 100g
Calories: 484 per 100g

**Bulgur Wheat Cereal:**
GI: Low to medium
GL: Low
Sugar: 0g (unsweetened)
Carbohydrates: 19g per 100g (cooked)
Calories: 83 per 100g (cooked)

**Chia Seed Pudding (No Added Sugar):**
GI: Low to medium
GL: Low
Sugar: 0g (unsweetened)
Carbohydrates: 9.8g per 100g (prepared)
Calories: 137 per 100g (prepared)

**Hemp Seed Cereal:**
GI: Low
GL: Low
Sugar: 1g per 100g
Carbohydrates: 5g per 100g
Calories: 360 per 100g

**Sunflower Seed Granola:**
GI: Low
GL: Low
Sugar: 6g per 100g
Carbohydrates: 44g per 100g
Calories: 450 per 100g

**Pearled Barley Cereal:**
GI: Low to medium
GL: Low
Sugar: 0g (unsweetened)
Carbohydrates: 28g per 100g (cooked)
Calories: 122 per 100g (cooked)

**Spelt Flakes:**
GI: Low to medium
GL: Low
Sugar: 0g (unsweetened)
Carbohydrates: 24g per 100g (cooked)
Calories: 123 per 100g (cooked)

**Millet Cereal:**
GI: Low to medium
GL: Low
Sugar: 1g per 100g (cooked)
Carbohydrates: 19g per 100g (cooked)
Calories: 119 per 100g (cooked)

**Pumpkin Seed Granola:**
GI: Low
GL: Low
Sugar: 6g per 100g
Carbohydrates: 45g per 100g
Calories: 480 per 100g

**Whole Grain Rye Flakes:**
GI: Low to medium
GL: Low
Sugar: 0g (unsweetened)
Carbohydrates: 28g per 100g (cooked)
Calories: 118 per 100g (cooked)

**Whole Wheat Cereal (Unsweetened):**
GI: Low to medium
GL: Low
Sugar: 0g (unsweetened)
Carbohydrates: 19g per 100g
Calories: 336 per 100g

**Black Rice Cereal:**
GI: Low
GL: Low
Sugar: 0g (unsweetened)
Carbohydrates: 22g per 100g (cooked)
Calories: 111 per 100g (cooked)

**Sorghum Flakes:**
GI: Low to medium
GL: Low
Sugar: 1g per 100g (cooked)
Carbohydrates: 20g per 100g (cooked)
Calories: 102 per 100g (cooked)

**Coconut Flour Cereal:**
GI: Low
GL: Low
Sugar: 2g per 100g
Carbohydrates: 35g per 100g
Calories: 450 per 100g

**Wild Rice Cereal:**
GI: Low to medium
GL: Low
Sugar: 0g (unsweetened)
Carbohydrates: 18g per 100g (cooked)
Calories: 101 per 100g (cooked)

**Whole Grain Teff Cereal:**
GI: Low
GL: Low
Sugar: 0g (unsweetened)
Carbohydrates: 19g per 100g (cooked)
Calories: 101 per 100g (cooked)

**Whole Grain Kamut Flakes:**
GI: Low to medium
GL: Low
Sugar: 0g (unsweetened)
Carbohydrates: 29g per 100g (cooked)
Calories: 122 per 100g (cooked)

**Bircher Muesli (No Added Sugar):**
GI: Low to medium
GL: Low
Sugar: 5g per 100g
Carbohydrates: 63g per 100g
Calories: 350 per 100g

## Legumes and Nuts

**Legumes:**
Lentils (Cooked):
GI: Low
GL: Low
Sugar: 2g per 100g
Carbohydrates: 20g per 100g
Calories: 116 per 100g

**Chickpeas (Cooked):**
GI: Low
GL: Low
Sugar: 4g per 100g
Carbohydrates: 27g per 100g
Calories: 164 per 100g

**Black Beans (Cooked):**
GI: Low
GL: Low
Sugar: 0g
Carbohydrates: 22g per 100g
Calories: 132 per 100g

**Kidney Beans (Cooked):**
GI: Low
GL: Low
Sugar: 0g
Carbohydrates: 22g per 100g
Calories: 127 per 100g

**Cannellini Beans (Cooked):**
GI: Low
GL: Low
Sugar: 0g
Carbohydrates: 20g per 100g
Calories: 120 per 100g

**Pinto Beans (Cooked):**
GI: Low
GL: Low
Sugar: 0g
Carbohydrates: 21g per 100g
Calories: 143 per 100g

**Green Peas (Cooked):**
GI: Low
GL: Low
Sugar: 6g per 100g
Carbohydrates: 14g per 100g
Calories: 81 per 100g

**Edamame (Cooked):**
GI: Low
GL: Low
Sugar: 2g per 100g
Carbohydrates: 8g per 100g
Calories: 122 per 100g

**Lima Beans (Cooked):**
GI: Low
GL: Low
Sugar: 1g per 100g
Carbohydrates: 19g per 100g
Calories: 115 per 100g

**Split Peas (Cooked):**
GI: Low
GL: Low
Sugar: 1g per 100g
Carbohydrates: 20g per 100g
Calories: 116 per 100g

**Adzuki Beans (Cooked):**
GI: Low
GL: Low
Sugar: 1g per 100g
Carbohydrates: 19g per 100g
Calories: 128 per 100g

**Black-Eyed Peas (Cooked):**
GI: Low
GL: Low
Sugar: 2g per 100g
Carbohydrates: 23g per 100g
Calories: 94 per 100g

# Nuts:

**Almonds:**
GI: Low
GL: Low
Sugar: 1g per 28g (23 almonds)
Carbohydrates: 6g per 28g
Calories: 160 per 28g

**Walnuts:**
GI: Low
GL: Low
Sugar: 1g per 28g (14 halves)
Carbohydrates: 4g per 28g
Calories: 185 per 28g

**Cashews:**
GI: Low
GL: Low
Sugar: 1g per 28g (18 nuts)
Carbohydrates: 9g per 28g
Calories: 155 per 28g

**Pistachios:**
GI: Low
GL: Low
Sugar: 2g per 28g (49 kernels)
Carbohydrates: 8g per 28g
Calories: 160 per 28g

**Brazil Nuts:**
GI: Low
GL: Low
Sugar: 0g per 28g (6 nuts)
Carbohydrates: 3g per 28g
Calories: 186 per 28g

**Hazelnuts:**
GI: Low
GL: Low
Sugar: 1g per 28g (21 nuts)
Carbohydrates: 5g per 28g
Calories: 180 per 28g

**Pecans:**
GI: Low
GL: Low
Sugar: 0g per 28g (19 halves)
Carbohydrates: 4g per 28g
Calories: 200 per 28g

**Macadamia Nuts:**
GI: Low
GL: Low
Sugar: 1g per 28g (10-12 nuts)
Carbohydrates: 4g per 28g
Calories: 200 per 28g

**Pine Nuts:**
GI: Low
GL: Low
Sugar: 1g per 28g (167 nuts)
Carbohydrates: 4g per 28g
Calories: 190 per 28g

**Sunflower Seeds:**
GI: Low
GL: Low
Sugar: 1g per 28g (1 oz)
Carbohydrates: 6g per 28g
Calories: 160 per 28g

**Chia Seeds:**
GI: Low
GL: Low
Sugar: 0g per 28g (2 tbsp)
Carbohydrates: 12g per 28g
Calories: 140 per 28g

**Flaxseeds:**
GI: Low
GL: Low
Sugar: 0g per 28g (2 tbsp)
Carbohydrates: 8g per 28g
Calories: 150 per 28g

**Sesame Seeds:**
GI: Low
GL: Low
Sugar: 0g per 28g (2 tbsp)
Carbohydrates: 6g per 28g
Calories: 160 per 28g

**Pumpkin Seeds:**
GI: Low
GL: Low
Sugar: 0g per 28g (1 oz)
Carbohydrates: 5g per 28g
Calories: 150 per 28g

**Poppy Seeds:**
GI: Low
GL: Low
Sugar: 0g per 28g (2 tbsp)
Carbohydrates: 6g per 28g
Calories: 100 per 28g

**Quinoa (Pseudocereal, but often considered a nut-like seed):**
GI: Low
GL: Low
Sugar: 0g per 185g (1 cup, cooked)
Carbohydrates: 39g per 185g (1 cup, cooked)
Calories: 222 per 185g (1 cup, cooked)

**Chestnuts**:
GI: Low
GL: Low
Sugar: 4g per 100g
Carbohydrates: 45g per 100g
Calories: 213 per 100g

**Soy Nuts (Roasted Soybeans):**
GI: Low
GL: Low
Sugar: 1g per 28g (1 oz)
Carbohydrates: 10g per 28g
Calories: 120 per 28g

# Milk and Alternatives:

### Whole Milk:
GI: Low
GL: Low
Sugar: 12g per cup
Carbohydrates: 12g per cup
Calories: 150 per cup

### Greek Yogurt (Full-fat, Unsweetened):
GI: Low
GL: Low
Sugar: 7g per 6 oz
Carbohydrates: 7g per 6 oz
Calories: 150 per 6 oz

### Cottage Cheese (Full-fat):
GI: Low
GL: Low
Sugar: 2g per half cup
Carbohydrates: 3g per half cup
Calories: 206 per half cup

### Buttermilk:
GI: Low
GL: Low
Sugar: 11g per cup
Carbohydrates: 12g per cup
Calories: 98 per cup

**Kefir (Unsweetened):**
GI: Low
GL: Low
Sugar: 0g (varies by fermentation time)
Carbohydrates: 12g per cup
Calories: 100 per cup

## Cheeses:

**Cheddar Cheese:**
GI: Low
GL: Low
Sugar: 0g
Carbohydrates: 1g per ounce
Calories: 115 per ounce

**Swiss Cheese:**
GI: Low
GL: Low
Sugar: 0g
Carbohydrates: 1g per slice (about 1 oz)
Calories: 106 per slice

**Feta Cheese:**
GI: Low
GL: Low
Sugar: 1g per ounce
Carbohydrates: 1g per ounce
Calories: 74 per ounce

**Mozzarella Cheese:**
GI: Low
GL: Low
Sugar: 0g
Carbohydrates: 1g per ounce
Calories: 85 per ounce

**Blue Cheese**:
GI: Low
GL: Low
Sugar: 0g
Carbohydrates: 1g per tablespoon
Calories: 100 per tablespoon

# Yogurts and Yogurt-Based Products:

**Skim Milk Yogurt (Unsweetened):**
GI: Low
GL: Low
Sugar: 9g per cup
Carbohydrates: 17g per cup
Calories: 137 per cup

**Probiotic Yogurt (Unsweetened):**
GI: Low
GL: Low
Sugar: 4g per cup
Carbohydrates: 11g per cup
Calories: 61 per cup

**Labneh (Strained Yogurt):**
GI: Low
GL: Low
Sugar: 2g per tablespoon
Carbohydrates: 3g per tablespoon
Calories: 50 per tablespoon

**Bulgarian Yogurt (Full-fat, Unsweetened):**
GI: Low
GL: Low
Sugar: 6g per cup
Carbohydrates: 7g per cup
Calories: 149 per cup

## Other Dairy Products:

**Butter:**
GI: Low
GL: Low
Sugar: 0g
Carbohydrates: 0g
Calories: 102 per tablespoon

**Sour Cream (Full-fat):**
GI: Low
GL: Low
Sugar: 1g per tablespoon
Carbohydrates: 1g per tablespoon
Calories: 52 per tablespoon

**Cream Cheese:**
GI: Low
GL: Low
Sugar: 1g per tablespoon
Carbohydrates: 1g per tablespoon
Calories: 51 per tablespoon

**Ghee:**
GI: Low
GL: Low
Sugar: 0g
Carbohydrates: 0g
Calories: 112 per tablespoon

**Mascarpone Cheese:**
GI: Low
GL: Low
Sugar: 0.1g per tablespoon
Carbohydrates: 0.2g per tablespoon
Calories: 50 per tablespoon

**Whole Milk Ricotta Cheese:**
GI: Low
GL: Low
Sugar: 3g per 4 oz
Carbohydrates: 3g per 4 oz
Calories: 330 per 4 oz

**Whole Milk:**
GI: Low
GL: Low
Sugar: 12g per cup
Carbohydrates: 12g per cup
Calories: 149 per cup

**Condensed Milk (Unsweetened):**
GI: Low
GL: Low
Sugar: 0g
Carbohydrates: 21g per cup
Calories: 982 per cup

**Evaporated Milk (Whole):**
GI: Low
GL: Low
Sugar: 11g per cup
Carbohydrates: 16g per cup
Calories: 338 per cup

**Creme Fraiche:**
GI: Low
GL: Low
Sugar: 0.6g per tablespoon
Carbohydrates: 0.6g per tablespoon
Calories: 51 per tablespoon

**Clotted Cream:**
GI: Low
GL: Low
Sugar: 0g
Carbohydrates: 0g
Calories: 684 per 100g

**Kokum Butter**:
GI: Low
GL: Low
Sugar: 0g
Carbohydrates: 0g
Calories: 862 per 100g

**Shea Butter:**
GI: Low
GL: Low
Sugar: 0g
Carbohydrates: 0g
Calories: 884 per 100g

**Milk Chocolate (High Cocoa Percentage):**
GI: Low to medium
GL: Low
Sugar: Varies
Carbohydrates: Varies
Calories: Varies

**Dark Chocolate (High Cocoa Percentage):**
GI: Low to medium
GL: Low
Sugar: Varies
Carbohydrates: Varies
Calories: Varies

**Cream (Heavy Whipping):**
GI: Low
GL: Low
Sugar: 0.5g per tablespoon
Carbohydrates: 0.5g per tablespoon
Calories: 52 per tablespoon

## Condiments, oil, fats

**Condiments:**
**Mustard:**
Sugar: 0g
Carbohydrates: 0g
Calories: 3 per teaspoon

**Hot Sauce (e.g., Tabasco):**
Sugar: 0g
Carbohydrates: 0g
Calories: 0 per teaspoon

**Soy Sauce (Reduced Sodium):**
Sugar: 1g per tablespoon
Carbohydrates: 1g per tablespoon
Calories: 10 per tablespoon

**Vinegar (White or Apple Cider):**
Sugar: 0g
Carbohydrates: 0g
Calories: 3 per tablespoon

**Salsa (No Added Sugar):**
Sugar: 4g per half cup
Carbohydrates: 7g per half cup
Calories: 30 per half cup

**Pesto Sauce:**
Sugar: 0.5g per tablespoon
Carbohydrates: 1g per tablespoon
Calories: 80 per tablespoon

**Worcestershire Sauce:**
Sugar: 1g per tablespoon
Carbohydrates: 1g per tablespoon
Calories: 15 per tablespoon

**Mayonnaise (Full-fat, No Sugar Added):**
Sugar: 0g
Carbohydrates: 0g
Calories: 94 per tablespoon

**Guacamole (Homemade, No Added Sugar):**
Sugar: 1g per tablespoon
Carbohydrates: 2g per tablespoon
Calories: 23 per tablespoon

**Horseradish Sauce:**
Sugar: 0.5g per teaspoon
Carbohydrates: 1g per teaspoon
Calories: 3 per teaspoon

## Oils:
**Olive Oil:**
Sugar: 0g
Carbohydrates: 0g
Calories: 119 per tablespoon

**Coconut Oil:**
Sugar: 0g
Carbohydrates: 0g
Calories: 117 per tablespoon

**Avocado Oil:**
Sugar: 0g
Carbohydrates: 0g
Calories: 124 per tablespoon

**Flaxseed Oil:**
Sugar: 0g
Carbohydrates: 0g
Calories: 120 per tablespoon

**Sesame Oil:**
Sugar: 0g
Carbohydrates: 0g
Calories: 120 per tablespoon

**Ghee:**
Sugar: 0g
Carbohydrates: 0g
Calories: 112 per tablespoon

**Walnut Oil:**
Sugar: 0g
Carbohydrates: 0g
Calories: 120 per tablespoon

**Peanut Oil:**
Sugar: 0g
Carbohydrates: 0g
Calories: 119 per tablespoon

**Sunflower Oil:**
Sugar: 0g
Carbohydrates: 0g
Calories: 124 per tablespoon

**Canola Oil:**
Sugar: 0g
Carbohydrates: 0g
Calories: 124 per tablespoon

**Fats:**
Butter (Unsalted):
Sugar: 0g
Carbohydrates: 0g
Calories: 102 per tablespoon

**Lard:**
Sugar: 0g
Carbohydrates: 0g
Calories: 115 per tablespoon

**Duck Fat:**
Sugar: 0g
Carbohydrates: 0g
Calories: 112 per tablespoon

**Bacon Grease:**
Sugar: 0g
Carbohydrates: 0g
Calories: 115 per tablespoon

**Chicken Fat (Schmaltz):**
Sugar: 0g
Carbohydrates: 0g
Calories: 115 per tablespoon

**Beef Tallow:**
Sugar: 0g
Carbohydrates: 0g
Calories: 115 per tablespoon

**Cocoa Butter:**
Sugar: 0g
Carbohydrates: 0g
Calories: 115 per tablespoon

**MCT Oil (Medium-Chain Triglyceride):**
Sugar: 0g
Carbohydrates: 0g
Calories: 130 per tablespoon

**Schmaltz (Rendered Chicken Fat):**
Sugar: 0g
Carbohydrates: 0g
Calories: 115 per tablespoon

**Grapeseed Oil:**
Sugar: 0g
Carbohydrates: 0g
Calories: 120 per tablespoon

**Cereals:**
***Steel-Cut Oats:***
GI: Low
GL: Low
Sugar: 0g per 100g (dry)
Carbohydrates: 62g per 100g (dry)
Calories: 379 per 100g (dry)

**Quinoa Flakes:**
GI: Low
GL: Low
Sugar: 0g per 100g (dry)
Carbohydrates: 64g per 100g (dry)
Calories: 368 per 100g (dry)

**Buckwheat Groats:**
GI: Low
GL: Low
Sugar: 1g per 100g (cooked)
Carbohydrates: 19g per 100g (cooked)
Calories: 92 per 100g (cooked)

**Amaranth:**
GI: Low
GL: Low
Sugar: 1g per 100g (cooked)
Carbohydrates: 19g per 100g (cooked)
Calories: 102 per 100g (cooked)

**Millet:**
GI: Low
GL: Low
Sugar: 0g per 100g (cooked)
Carbohydrates: 23g per 100g (cooked)
Calories: 119 per 100g (cooked)

**Barley (Pearl, cooked):**
GI: Low to medium
GL: Low
Sugar: 0g per 100g (cooked)
Carbohydrates: 14g per 100g (cooked)
Calories: 96 per 100g (cooked)

**Brown Rice (Basmati, cooked):**
GI: Low
GL: Low
Sugar: 0g per 100g (cooked)
Carbohydrates: 23g per 100g (cooked)
Calories: 111 per 100g (cooked)

**Wild Rice:**
GI: Low
GL: Low
Sugar: 0g per 100g (cooked)
Carbohydrates: 21g per 100g (cooked)
Calories: 101 per 100g (cooked)

**Bran Flakes:**
GI: Low to medium
GL: Low
Sugar: 8g per 100g
Carbohydrates: 58g per 100g
Calories: 343 per 100g

**Kamut Flakes:**
GI: Low
GL: Low
Sugar: 0g per 100g
Carbohydrates: 14g per 100g
Calories: 66 per 100g

**Rice:**

**Basmati Rice (Brown, cooked):**
GI: Low
GL: Low
Sugar: 0g per 100g (cooked)
Carbohydrates: 22g per 100g (cooked)
Calories: 123 per 100g (cooked)

**Jasmine Rice (Brown, cooked):**
GI: Low
GL: Low
Sugar: 0g per 100g (cooked)
Carbohydrates: 23g per 100g (cooked)
Calories: 111 per 100g (cooked)

**Parboiled Rice:**
GI: Low
GL: Low
Sugar: 0g per 100g (cooked)
Carbohydrates: 23g per 100g (cooked)
Calories: 121 per 100g (cooked)

**Red Rice:**
GI: Low to medium
GL: Low
Sugar: 0g per 100g (cooked)
Carbohydrates: 23g per 100g (cooked)
Calories: 123 per 100g (cooked)

**Black Rice:**
GI: Low to medium
GL: Low
Sugar: 0g per 100g (cooked)
Carbohydrates: 23g per 100g (cooked)
Calories: 111 per 100g (cooked)

**Grains:**

**Freekeh:**
GI: Low
GL: Low
Sugar: 0g per 100g (cooked)
Carbohydrates: 16g per 100g (cooked)
Calories: 143 per 100g (cooked)

**Sorghum:**
GI: Low
GL: Low
Sugar: 0g per 100g (cooked)
Carbohydrates: 24g per 100g (cooked)
Calories: 101 per 100g (cooked)

**Spelt (cooked):**
GI: Low
GL: Low
Sugar: 0g per 100g (cooked)
Carbohydrates: 15g per 100g (cooked)
Calories: 120 per 100g (cooked)

**Teff:**
GI: Low
GL: Low
Sugar: 0g per 100g (cooked)
Carbohydrates: 20g per 100g (cooked)
Calories: 101 per 100g (cooked)

**Einkorn:**
GI: Low
GL: Low
Sugar: 0g per 100g (cooked)
Carbohydrates: 14g per 100g (cooked)
Calories: 83 per 100g (cooked)

**Additional Grains:**

**Muesli (No Added Sugar):**
GI: Low to medium
GL: Low
Sugar: 5g per 100g
Carbohydrates: 63g per 100g
Calories: 350 per 100g

**Bulgur Wheat (cooked):**
GI: Low to medium
GL: Low
Sugar: 0g per 100g (cooked)
Carbohydrates: 18g per 100g (cooked)
Calories: 76 per 100g (cooked)

**Whole Wheat Couscous (cooked):**
GI: Low to medium
GL: Low
Sugar: 0g per 100g (cooked)
Carbohydrates: 23g per 100g (cooked)
Calories: 112 per 100g (cooked)

**Rye Berries (cooked):**
GI: Low
GL: Low
Sugar: 0g per 100g (cooked)
Carbohydrates: 21g per 100g (cooked)
Calories: 83 per 100g (cooked)

**Soba Noodles (Buckwheat):**
GI: Low to medium
GL: Low
Sugar: 0g per 100g (cooked)
Carbohydrates: 21g per 100g (cooked)
Calories: 99 per 100g (cooked)

**Granola and Muesli:**

**Granola (No Added Sugar):**
GI: Low to medium
GL: Low
Sugar: 5g per 100g
Carbohydrates: 64g per 100g
Calories: 410 per 100g

**Oat Bran:**
GI: Low
GL: Low
Sugar: 1g per 100g (raw)
Carbohydrates: 66g per 100g (raw)
Calories: 246 per 100g (raw)

**Bran Flakes:**
GI: Low to medium
GL: Low
Sugar: 8g per 100g
Carbohydrates: 58g per 100g
Calories: 343 per 100g

**Wheat Germ:**
GI: Low
GL: Low
Sugar: 1g per 100g
Carbohydrates: 50g per 100g
Calories: 382 per 100g

**Grape Nuts (No Added Sugar):**
GI: Low to medium
GL: Low
Sugar: 7g per 100g
Carbohydrates: 76g per 100g
Calories: 366 per 100g

**Basil:**
Carbohydrates: 2g per 100g
Calories: 23 per 100g

**Cilantro (Coriander):**
Carbohydrates: 3g per 100g
Calories: 23 per 100g

**Mint:**
Carbohydrates: 14g per 100g
Calories: 70 per 100g

**Parsley:**
Carbohydrates: 6g per 100g
Calories: 36 per 100g

**Chives:**
Carbohydrates: 4g per 100g
Calories: 30 per 100g

**Dill:**
Carbohydrates: 7g per 100g
Calories: 43 per 100g

**Thyme:**
Carbohydrates: 24g per 100g
Calories: 101 per 100g

**Rosemary:**
Carbohydrates: 21g per 100g
Calories: 131 per 100g

**Sage:**
Carbohydrates: 26g per 100g
Calories: 43 per 100g

**Oregano:**
Carbohydrates: 27g per 100g
Calories: 265 per 100g

**Cilantro (Coriander) Leaves:**
Carbohydrates: 3g per 100g
Calories: 23 per 100g

**Parsley Leaves:**
Carbohydrates: 6g per 100g
Calories: 36 per 100g

**Chives (Raw):**
Carbohydrates: 4g per 100g
Calories: 30 per 100g

**Basil (Fresh Leaves):**
Carbohydrates: 2g per 100g
Calories: 23 per 100g

**Mint Leaves:**
Carbohydrates: 14g per 100g
Calories: 70 per 100g

**Cilantro (Coriander) Roots:**
Carbohydrates: 8g per 100g
Calories: 23 per 100g

**Dill Leaves:**
Carbohydrates: 7g per 100g
Calories: 43 per 100g

**Thyme (Fresh):**
Carbohydrates: 24g per 100g
Calories: 101 per 100g

**Rosemary (Fresh):**
Carbohydrates: 21g per 100g
Calories: 131 per 100g

**Sage Leaves:**
Carbohydrates: 26g per 100g
Calories: 43 per 100g

**Oregano (Fresh Leaves):**
Carbohydrates: 27g per 100g
Calories: 265 per 100g

**Tarragon:**
Carbohydrates: 50g per 100g
Calories: 295 per 100g


**Lemon Balm:**
Carbohydrates: 25g per 100g
Calories: 43 per 100g


**Culantro (Mexican Coriander):**
Carbohydrates: 2g per 100g
Calories: 22 per 100g


**Lavender:**
Carbohydrates: 29g per 100g
Calories: 100 per 100g


**Marjoram:**
Carbohydrates: 43g per 100g
Calories: 271 per 100g


**Chervil:**
Carbohydrates: 35g per 100g
Calories: 237 per 100g


**Lovage:**
Carbohydrates: 37g per 100g
Calories: 22 per 100g

**Coriander Seeds:**
Carbohydrates: 54g per 100g
Calories: 298 per 100g

**Fennel Fronds:**
Carbohydrates: 7g per 100g
Calories: 31 per 100g

## Legumes

**Lentils (Green, Cooked):**
GI: Low
GL: Low
Sugar: 2g per 100g
Carbohydrates: 20g per 100g
Calories: 116 per 100g

**Chickpeas (Garbanzo Beans, Cooked):**
GI: Low
GL: Low
Sugar: 4g per 100g
Carbohydrates: 27g per 100g
Calories: 164 per 100g

**Black Beans (Cooked):**
GI: Low
GL: Low
Sugar: 0g per 100g
Carbohydrates: 22g per 100g
Calories: 120 per 100g

**Kidney Beans (Cooked):**
GI: Low
GL: Low
Sugar: 0g per 100g
Carbohydrates: 22g per 100g
Calories: 127 per 100g

**Cannellini Beans (Cooked):**
GI: Low
GL: Low
Sugar: 0g per 100g
Carbohydrates: 20g per 100g
Calories: 100 per 100g

**Pinto Beans (Cooked):**
GI: Low
GL: Low
Sugar: 0g per 100g
Carbohydrates: 21g per 100g
Calories: 123 per 100g

**Adzuki Beans (Cooked):**
GI: Low
GL: Low
Sugar: 0g per 100g
Carbohydrates: 19g per 100g
Calories: 128 per 100g

**Black-Eyed Peas (Cooked):**
GI: Low
GL: Low
Sugar: 0g per 100g
Carbohydrates: 23g per 100g
Calories: 120 per 100g

**Mung Beans (Cooked):**
GI: Low
GL: Low
Sugar: 1g per 100g
Carbohydrates: 14g per 100g
Calories: 105 per 100g

**Split Peas (Cooked):**
GI: Low
GL: Low
Sugar: 1g per 100g
Carbohydrates: 20g per 100g
Calories: 116 per 100g

**Lima Beans (Cooked):**
GI: Low
GL: Low
Sugar: 2g per 100g
Carbohydrates: 19g per 100g
Calories: 115 per 100g

**Navy Beans (Cooked):**
GI: Low
GL: Low
Sugar: 0g per 100g
Carbohydrates: 19g per 100g
Calories: 127 per 100g

**Great Northern Beans (Cooked):**
GI: Low
GL: Low
Sugar: 0g per 100g
Carbohydrates: 19g per 100g
Calories: 100 per 100g

**Fava Beans (Cooked):**
GI: Low
GL: Low
Sugar: 0g per 100g
Carbohydrates: 26g per 100g
Calories: 110 per 100g

**Chana Dal (Split Chickpeas, Cooked):**
GI: Low
GL: Low
Sugar: 4g per 100g
Carbohydrates: 27g per 100g
Calories: 160 per 100g

**Yellow Split Peas (Cooked):**
GI: Low
GL: Low
Sugar: 2g per 100g
Carbohydrates: 20g per 100g
Calories: 116 per 100g

**Green Peas (Cooked):**
GI: Low
GL: Low
Sugar: 5g per 100g
Carbohydrates: 14g per 100g
Calories: 81 per 100g

**Cowpeas (Black-Eyed Peas, Cooked):**
GI: Low
GL: Low
Sugar: 0g per 100g
Carbohydrates: 24g per 100g
Calories: 118 per 100g

**Chickpea Flour (Besan):**
GI: Low
GL: Low
Sugar: 10g per 100g
Carbohydrates: 58g per 100g
Calories: 387 per 100g

**Lentil Soup (Canned):**
GI: Low
GL: Low
Sugar: 3g per 100g
Carbohydrates: 14g per 100g
Calories: 83 per 100g

**Refried Beans (Canned):**
GI: Low
GL: Low
Sugar: 1g per 100g
Carbohydrates: 19g per 100g
Calories: 91 per 100g

**Black Bean Soup (Canned):**
GI: Low
GL: Low
Sugar: 1g per 100g
Carbohydrates: 15g per 100g
Calories: 82 per 100g

**Lentil Patties (Cooked):**
GI: Low
GL: Low
Sugar: 2g per 100g
Carbohydrates: 20g per 100g
Calories: 116 per 100g

**Hummus:**
GI: Low
GL: Low
Sugar: 0g per 100g
Carbohydrates: 18g per 100g
Calories: 166 per 100g

**Edamame (Cooked):**
GI: Low
GL: Low
Sugar: 2g per 100g
Carbohydrates: 8g per 100g
Calories: 121 per 100g

**Pea Soup (Canned):**
GI: Low
GL: Low
Sugar: 1g per 100g
Carbohydrates: 12g per 100g
Calories: 77 per 100g

**Chickpea Salad:**
GI: Low
GL: Low
Sugar: 2g per 100g
Carbohydrates: 14g per 100g
Calories: 81 per 100g

**White Bean Soup (Canned):**
GI: Low
GL: Low
Sugar: 1g per 100g
Carbohydrates: 17g per 100g
Calories: 83 per 100g

**Red Lentils (Cooked):**
GI: Low
GL: Low
Sugar: 1g per 100g
Carbohydrates: 20g per 100g
Calories: 116 per 100g

*Green Split Peas (Cooked):*
GI: Low
GL: Low
Sugar: 1g per 100g
Carbohydrates: 20g per 100g
Calories: 116 per 100g

**Whole Wheat Bread:**
GI: Low to medium
GL: Low
Sugar: 2g per slice
Carbohydrates: 12g per slice
Calories: 69 per slice

**Multigrain Bread:**
GI: Low to medium
GL: Low
Sugar: 3g per slice
Carbohydrates: 14g per slice
Calories: 80 per slice

**Rye Bread**:
GI: Low
GL: Low
Sugar: 1g per slice
Carbohydrates: 15g per slice
Calories: 83 per slice

**Pumpernickel Bread:**
GI: Low
GL: Low
Sugar: 1g per slice
Carbohydrates: 15g per slice
Calories: 80 per slice

**Sprouted Grain Bread:**
GI: Low
GL: Low
Sugar: 0g per slice
Carbohydrates: 15g per slice
Calories: 60 per slice

**Barley Bread:**
GI: Low to medium
GL: Low
Sugar: 1g per slice
Carbohydrates: 15g per slice
Calories: 74 per slice

**Oat Bran Bread:**
GI: Low to medium
GL: Low
Sugar: 2g per slice
Carbohydrates: 15g per slice
Calories: 70 per slice

**Quinoa Bread:**
GI: Low to medium
GL: Low
Sugar: 1g per slice
Carbohydrates: 14g per slice
Calories: 70 per slice

**Sourdough Bread:**

GI: Low
GL: Low
Sugar: 0g per slice
Carbohydrates: 12g per slice
Calories: 68 per slice

**Whole Grain Spelt Bread:**

GI: Low to medium
GL: Low
Sugar: 2g per slice
Carbohydrates: 15g per slice
Calories: 80 per slice

**Ezekiel Bread:**

GI: Low
GL: Low
Sugar: 0g per slice
Carbohydrates: 15g per slice
Calories: 80 per slice

**Buckwheat Bread:**

GI: Low
GL: Low
Sugar: 1g per slice
Carbohydrates: 15g per slice
Calories: 80 per slice

**Brown Rice Bread:**
GI: Low to medium
GL: Low
Sugar: 1g per slice
Carbohydrates: 15g per slice
Calories: 70 per slice

**Hemp Bread:**
GI: Low to medium
GL: Low
Sugar: 1g per slice
Carbohydrates: 15g per slice
Calories: 80 per slice

**Amaranth Bread:**
GI: Low to medium
GL: Low
Sugar: 1g per slice
Carbohydrates: 14g per slice
Calories: 70 per slice

**Teff Bread:**
GI: Low
GL: Low
Sugar: 1g per slice
Carbohydrates: 15g per slice
Calories: 70 per slice

**Sweet Potato Bread:**

GI: Low to medium

GL: Low

Sugar: 2g per slice

Carbohydrates: 15g per slice

Calories: 80 per slice

**Chickpea Flour Bread:**

GI: Low to medium

GL: Low

Sugar: 1g per slice

Carbohydrates: 15g per slice

Calories: 70 per slice

**Coconut Flour Bread**:

GI: Low

GL: Low

Sugar: 1g per slice

Carbohydrates: 10g per slice

Calories: 70 per slice

**Almond Flour Bread:**

GI: Low

GL: Low

Sugar: 0g per slice

Carbohydrates: 1g per slice

Calories: 40 per slice

**Flaxseed Bread:**
GI: Low
GL: Low
Sugar: 1g per slice
Carbohydrates: 12g per slice
Calories: 60 per slice

**Hazelnut Bread:**
GI: Low
GL: Low
Sugar: 1g per slice
Carbohydrates: 12g per slice
Calories: 60 per slice

**Millet Bread:**
GI: Low to medium
GL: Low
Sugar: 2g per slice
Carbohydrates: 15g per slice
Calories: 80 per slice

**Cauliflower Bread:**
GI: Low
GL: Low
Sugar: 1g per slice
Carbohydrates: 5g per slice
Calories: 50 per slice

**Sunflower Seed Bread:**

GI: Low to medium

GL: Low

Sugar: 1g per slice

Carbohydrates: 12g per slice

Calories: 60 per slice

**Pistachio Bread:**

GI: Low

GL: Low

Sugar: 1g per slice

Carbohydrates: 12g per slice

Calories: 60 per slice

**Sesame Seed Bread:**

GI: Low

GL: Low

Sugar: 1g per slice

Carbohydrates: 12g per slice

Calories: 60 per slice

**Chestnut Flour Bread:**

GI: Low to medium

GL: Low

Sugar: 2g per slice

Carbohydrates: 15g per slice

Calories: 80 per slice

**Acorn Flour Bread:**
GI: Low
GL: Low
Sugar: 1g per slice
Carbohydrates: 12g per slice
Calories: 60 per slice

**Cassava Flour Bread:**
GI: Low to medium
GL: Low
Sugar: 2g per slice
Carbohydrates: 15g per slice
Calories: 80 per slice

## Canned foods

**Canned Black Beans:**
GI: Low
GL: Low
Sugar: 0g per half cup
Carbohydrates: 20g per half cup
Calories: 110 per half cup

**Canned Chickpeas:**
GI: Low
GL: Low
Sugar: 2g per half cup
Carbohydrates: 27g per half cup
Calories: 134 per half cup

**Canned Lentils:**
GI: Low
GL: Low
Sugar: 2g per half cup
Carbohydrates: 20g per half cup
Calories: 115 per half cup

**Canned Kidney Beans:**
GI: Low
GL: Low
Sugar: 1g per half cup
Carbohydrates: 22g per half cup
Calories: 112 per half cup

**Canned Green Beans:**
GI: Low
GL: Low
Sugar: 2g per half cup
Carbohydrates: 4g per half cup
Calories: 20 per half cup

**Canned Tomatoes:**
GI: Low
GL: Low
Sugar: 3g per half cup
Carbohydrates: 5g per half cup
Calories: 25 per half cup

**Canned Spinach:**
GI: Low
GL: Low
Sugar: 0g per half cup
Carbohydrates: 3g per half cup
Calories: 15 per half cup

**Canned Artichoke Hearts:**
GI: Low
GL: Low
Sugar: 1g per half cup
Carbohydrates: 4g per half cup
Calories: 25 per half cup

**Canned Asparagus:**
GI: Low
GL: Low
Sugar: 0g per half cup
Carbohydrates: 3g per half cup
Calories: 15 per half cup

**Canned Mushrooms**:
GI: Low
GL: Low
Sugar: 0g per half cup
Carbohydrates: 1g per half cup
Calories: 10 per half cup

**Canned Tuna in Water:**
GI: Low
GL: Low
Sugar: 0g per 3 ounces
Carbohydrates: 0g per 3 ounces
Calories: 100 per 3 ounces

**Canned Salmon:**
GI: Low
GL: Low
Sugar: 0g per 3 ounces
Carbohydrates: 0g per 3 ounces
Calories: 120 per 3 ounces

**Canned Sardines in Water:**
GI: Low
GL: Low
Sugar: 0g per 3 ounces
Carbohydrates: 0g per 3 ounces
Calories: 150 per 3 ounces

**Canned Chicken Breast:**
GI: Low
GL: Low
Sugar: 0g per 3 ounces
Carbohydrates: 0g per 3 ounces
Calories: 110 per 3 ounces

**Canned Pumpkin Puree:**
GI: Low
GL: Low
Sugar: 3g per half cup
Carbohydrates: 12g per half cup
Calories: 50 per half cup

**Canned Peas:**
GI: Low
GL: Low
Sugar: 5g per half cup
Carbohydrates: 12g per half cup
Calories: 65 per half cup

**Canned Carrots:**
GI: Low
GL: Low
Sugar: 4g per half cup
Carbohydrates: 10g per half cup
Calories: 45 per half cup

**Canned Beets:**
GI: Low to medium
GL: Low
Sugar: 6g per half cup
Carbohydrates: 16g per half cup
Calories: 75 per half cup

**Canned Sweet Potatoes:**
GI: Low to medium
GL: Low
Sugar: 6g per half cup
Carbohydrates: 16g per half cup
Calories: 90 per half cup

**Canned Green Peas:**
GI: Low
GL: Low
Sugar: 6g per half cup
Carbohydrates: 12g per half cup
Calories: 62 per half cup

**Canned Corn:**
GI: Low to medium
GL: Low
Sugar: 3g per half cup
Carbohydrates: 18g per half cup
Calories: 75 per half cup

**Canned Avocado (Unsweetened):**
GI: Low
GL: Low
Sugar: 0g per half cup
Carbohydrates: 4g per half cup
Calories: 120 per half cup

**Canned Brussels Sprouts:**
GI: Low
GL: Low
Sugar: 1g per half cup
Carbohydrates: 4g per half cup
Calories: 30 per half cup

**Canned Okra:**
GI: Low
GL: Low
Sugar: 1g per half cup
Carbohydrates: 4g per half cup
Calories: 25 per half cup

**Canned Zucchini:**
GI: Low
GL: Low
Sugar: 1g per half cup
Carbohydrates: 4g per half cup
Calories: 15 per half cup

**Canned Cranberry Sauce (Unsweetened):**
GI: Low to medium
GL: Low
Sugar: 4g per quarter cup
Carbohydrates: 11g per quarter cup
Calories: 50 per quarter cup

**Canned Green Chilies:**
GI: Low
GL: Low
Sugar: 2g per half cup
Carbohydrates: 4g per half cup
Calories: 20 per half cup

**Canned Eggplant:**
GI: Low
GL: Low
Sugar: 1g per half cup
Carbohydrates: 5g per half cup
Calories: 20 per half cup

**Canned Water Chestnuts:**
GI: Low
GL: Low
Sugar: 0g per half cup
Carbohydrates: 4g per half cup
Calories: 35 per half cup

**Canned Bamboo Shoots:**
GI: Low
GL: Low
Sugar: 0g per half cup
Carbohydrates: 2g per half cup
Calories: 20 per half cup

**Grilled Chicken Salad:**
GI: Low
GL: Low
Sugar: 2g per serving
Carbohydrates: 10g per serving
Calories: 200 per serving

**Salmon and Quinoa Bowl:**
GI: Low
GL: Low
Sugar: 3g per serving
Carbohydrates: 20g per serving
Calories: 300 per serving

**Vegetarian Stir-Fry with Tofu:**
GI: Low
GL: Low
Sugar: 4g per serving
Carbohydrates: 15g per serving
Calories: 250 per serving

**Shrimp and Vegetable Skewers:**
GI: Low
GL: Low
Sugar: 2g per serving
Carbohydrates: 12g per serving
Calories: 180 per serving

**Turkey and Avocado Wrap:**

GI: Low

GL: Low

Sugar: 2g per serving

Carbohydrates: 15g per serving

Calories: 220 per serving

**Egg and Spinach Breakfast Wrap:**

GI: Low

GL: Low

Sugar: 1g per serving

Carbohydrates: 10g per serving

Calories: 180 per serving

**Mushroom and Spinach Omelette:**

GI: Low

GL: Low

Sugar: 2g per serving

Carbohydrates: 8g per serving

Calories: 150 per serving

**Grilled Vegetable Quiche:**

GI: Low

GL: Low

Sugar: 3g per serving

Carbohydrates: 18g per serving

Calories: 250 per serving

**Chicken and Broccoli Stir-Fry with Brown Rice:**
GI: Low
GL: Low
Sugar: 4g per serving
Carbohydrates: 25g per serving
Calories: 280 per serving

**Caprese Salad with Balsamic Glaze:**
GI: Low
GL: Low
Sugar: 3g per serving
Carbohydrates: 10g per serving
Calories: 220 per serving

**Spaghetti Squash with Tomato Sauce and Turkey Meatballs**:
GI: Low
GL: Low
Sugar: 5g per serving
Carbohydrates: 20g per serving
Calories: 280 per serving

**Chickpea and Vegetable Curry:**
GI: Low
GL: Low
Sugar: 4g per serving
Carbohydrates: 30g per serving
Calories: 270 per serving

**Brown Rice and Black Bean Burrito Bowl:**

GI: Low

GL: Low

Sugar: 3g per serving

Carbohydrates: 25g per serving

Calories: 300 per serving

**Turkey and Sweet Potato Chili:**

GI: Low

GL: Low

Sugar: 4g per serving

Carbohydrates: 20g per serving

Calories: 280 per serving

**Quinoa and Roasted Vegetable Stuffed Bell Peppers:**

GI: Low

GL: Low

Sugar: 3g per serving

Carbohydrates: 25g per serving

Calories: 260 per serving

**Lentil Soup with Greens:**

GI: Low

GL: Low

Sugar: 2g per serving

Carbohydrates: 15g per serving

Calories: 180 per serving

**Cauliflower Fried Rice with Shrimp:**
GI: Low
GL: Low
Sugar: 3g per serving
Carbohydrates: 20g per serving
Calories: 240 per serving

**Greek Yogurt Parfait with Berries and Nuts**:
GI: Low
GL: Low
Sugar: 8g per serving
Carbohydrates: 20g per serving
Calories: 220 per serving

**Vegetable and Quinoa Stuffed Portobello Mushrooms:**
GI: Low
GL: Low
Sugar: 3g per serving
Carbohydrates: 18g per serving
Calories: 230 per serving

**Lemon Garlic Chicken with Roasted Brussels Sprouts:**
GI: Low
GL: Low
Sugar: 2g per serving
Carbohydrates: 15g per serving
Calories: 250 per serving

**Mediterranean Chickpea Salad:**

GI: Low

GL: Low

Sugar: 4g per serving

Carbohydrates: 20g per serving

Calories: 230 per serving

**Zucchini Noodles with Pesto and Cherry Tomatoes:**

GI: Low

GL: Low

Sugar: 3g per serving

Carbohydrates: 15g per serving

Calories: 210 per serving

**Cottage Cheese and Berry Bowl:**

GI: Low

GL: Low

Sugar: 10g per serving

Carbohydrates: 20g per serving

Calories: 180 per serving

**Quinoa Salad with Feta and Cucumber:**

GI: Low

GL: Low

Sugar: 4g per serving

Carbohydrates: 25g per serving

Calories: 260 per serving

**Shakshuka (Poached Eggs in Spicy Tomato Sauce):**
GI: Low
GL: Low
Sugar: 6g per serving
Carbohydrates: 15g per serving
Calories: 220 per serving

**Turkey and Vegetable Skillet:**
GI: Low
GL: Low
Sugar: 3g per serving
Carbohydrates: 20g per serving
Calories: 240 per serving

**Chia Seed Pudding with Almond Milk and Berries:**
GI: Low
GL: Low
Sugar: 8g per serving
Carbohydrates: 20g per serving
Calories: 180 per serving

**Stuffed Bell Peppers with Ground Turkey and Quinoa:**
GI: Low
GL: Low
Sugar: 4g per serving
Carbohydrates: 25g per serving
Calories: 270 per serving

**Chicken Caesar Salad with Kale:**
GI: Low
GL: Low
Sugar: 2g per serving
Carbohydrates: 12g per serving
Calories: 220 per serving

**Brown Rice Sushi Rolls with Avocado and Salmon:**
GI: Low to medium
GL: Low
Sugar: 3g per serving
Carbohydrates: 30g per serving
Calories: 280 per serving

## Pasta and Noodles

**Whole Wheat Pasta:**
GI: Low to medium
GL: Low
Sugar: 1g per 2 oz (uncooked)
Carbohydrates: 39g per 2 oz (uncooked)
Calories: 180 per 2 oz (uncooked)

**Brown Rice Pasta:**
GI: Low
GL: Low
Sugar: 0g per 2 oz (uncooked)
Carbohydrates: 43g per 2 oz (uncooked)
Calories: 200 per 2 oz (uncooked)

**Quinoa Pasta:**
GI: Low
GL: Low
Sugar: 1g per 2 oz (uncooked)
Carbohydrates: 42g per 2 oz (uncooked)
Calories: 200 per 2 oz (uncooked)

**Lentil Pasta:**
GI: Low
GL: Low
Sugar: 0g per 2 oz (uncooked)
Carbohydrates: 34g per 2 oz (uncooked)
Calories: 190 per 2 oz (uncooked)

**Chickpea Pasta:**
GI: Low
GL: Low
Sugar: 1g per 2 oz (uncooked)
Carbohydrates: 32g per 2 oz (uncooked)
Calories: 180 per 2 oz (uncooked)

**Buckwheat Noodles (Soba):**
GI: Low to medium
GL: Low
Sugar: 0g per 2 oz (cooked)
Carbohydrates: 36g per 2 oz (cooked)
Calories: 200 per 2 oz (cooked)

**Spelt Pasta:**
GI: Low to medium
GL: Low
Sugar: 1g per 2 oz (uncooked)
Carbohydrates: 38g per 2 oz (uncooked)
Calories: 200 per 2 oz (uncooked)

**Barley Noodles:**
GI: Low to medium
GL: Low
Sugar: 0g per 2 oz (uncooked)
Carbohydrates: 42g per 2 oz (uncooked)
Calories: 200 per 2 oz (uncooked)

**Artichoke Pasta:**
GI: Low
GL: Low
Sugar: 0g per 2 oz (uncooked)
Carbohydrates: 44g per 2 oz (uncooked)
Calories: 210 per 2 oz (uncooked)

**Shirataki Noodles:**
GI: Low
GL: Low
Sugar: 0g per serving
Carbohydrates: 1g per serving
Calories: 0 per serving

**Sweet Potato Noodles:**
GI: Low to medium
GL: Low
Sugar: 4g per 2 oz (uncooked)
Carbohydrates: 44g per 2 oz (uncooked)
Calories: 210 per 2 oz (uncooked)

**Konjac Noodles:**
GI: Low
GL: Low
Sugar: 0g per serving
Carbohydrates: 1g per serving
Calories: 5 per serving

**Einkorn Pasta:**
GI: Low to medium
GL: Low
Sugar: 1g per 2 oz (uncooked)
Carbohydrates: 40g per 2 oz (uncooked)
Calories: 190 per 2 oz (uncooked)

**Black Bean Pasta:**
GI: Low
GL: Low
Sugar: 1g per 2 oz (uncooked)
Carbohydrates: 30g per 2 oz (uncooked)
Calories: 180 per 2 oz (uncooked)

**Chestnut Flour Pasta:**
GI: Low to medium
GL: Low
Sugar: 1g per 2 oz (uncooked)
Carbohydrates: 42g per 2 oz (uncooked)
Calories: 200 per 2 oz (uncooked)

**Rice Noodles**:
GI: Low to medium
GL: Low
Sugar: 0g per 2 oz (cooked)
Carbohydrates: 41g per 2 oz (cooked)
Calories: 192 per 2 oz (cooked)

**Mung Bean Noodles**:
GI: Low
GL: Low
Sugar: 0g per 2 oz (cooked)
Carbohydrates: 36g per 2 oz (cooked)
Calories: 160 per 2 oz (cooked)

**Buckwheat Soba Noodles:**
GI: Low to medium
GL: Low
Sugar: 0g per 2 oz (cooked)
Carbohydrates: 33g per 2 oz (cooked)
Calories: 160 per 2 oz (cooked)

**Chia Seed Pasta:**
GI: Low
GL: Low
Sugar: 0g per 2 oz (uncooked)
Carbohydrates: 36g per 2 oz (uncooked)
Calories: 180 per 2 oz (uncooked)

**Sorghum Pasta:**
GI: Low
GL: Low
Sugar: 0g per 2 oz (uncooked)
Carbohydrates: 40g per 2 oz (uncooked)
Calories: 200 per 2 oz (uncooked)

**Rice Stick Noodles:**
GI: Low to medium
GL: Low
Sugar: 0g per 2 oz (cooked)
Carbohydrates: 40g per 2 oz (cooked)
Calories: 192 per 2 oz (cooked)

**Buckwheat Pancakes (as noodles substitute):**
GI: Low to medium
GL: Low
Sugar: 1g per pancake
Carbohydrates: 18g per pancake
Calories: 80 per pancake

**Cauliflower Gnocchi:**

GI: Low

GL: Low

Sugar: 2g per 1 cup (cooked)

Carbohydrates: 22g per 1 cup (cooked)

Calories: 140 per 1 cup (cooked)

**Almond Flour Pasta:**

GI: Low

GL: Low

Sugar: 1g per 2 oz (uncooked)

Carbohydrates: 22g per 2 oz (uncooked)

Calories: 200 per 2 oz (uncooked)

**Hemp Seed Pasta:**

GI: Low

GL: Low

Sugar: 1g per 2 oz (uncooked)

Carbohydrates: 36g per 2 oz (uncooked)

Calories: 200 per 2 oz (uncooked)

**Butternut Squash Noodles:**

GI: Low to medium

GL: Low

Sugar: 2g per 2 oz (uncooked)

Carbohydrates: 22g per 2 oz (uncooked)

Calories: 100 per 2 oz (uncooked)

**Chickpea Gnocchi:**
GI: Low
GL: Low
Sugar: 2g per 1 cup (cooked)
Carbohydrates: 32g per 1 cup (cooked)
Calories: 190 per 1 cup (cooked)

**Acorn Squash Pasta:**
GI: Low to medium
GL: Low
Sugar: 2g per 2 oz (uncooked)
Carbohydrates: 24g per 2 oz (uncooked)
Calories: 110 per 2 oz (uncooked)

**Edamame Pasta:**
GI: Low
GL: Low
Sugar: 0g per 2 oz (uncooked)
Carbohydrates: 13g per 2 oz (uncooked)
Calories: 180 per 2 oz (uncooked)

**Green Pea Pasta:**
GI: Low
GL: Low
Sugar: 0g per 2 oz (uncooked)
Carbohydrates: 22g per 2 oz (uncooked)
Calories: 190 per 2 oz (uncooked)

**Stevia (Natural Sweetener):**
GI: Low
GL: Low
Sugar: 0g per packet
Carbohydrates: 1g per packet
Calories: 0 per packet

**Monk Fruit Sweetener:**
GI: Low
GL: Low
Sugar: 0g per packet
Carbohydrates: 0g per packet
Calories: 0 per packet

**Erythritol (Sugar Alcohol):**
GI: Low
GL: Low
Sugar: 0g per teaspoon
Carbohydrates: 4g per teaspoon
Calories: 0.2 per gram

**Xylitol (Sugar Alcohol):**
GI: Low
GL: Low
Sugar: 0g per teaspoon
Carbohydrates: 4g per teaspoon
Calories: 2.4 per gram

**Agave Nectar (in moderation):**
GI: Low to medium
GL: Low
Sugar: 16g per tablespoon
Carbohydrates: 16g per tablespoon
Calories: 60 per tablespoon

**Coconut Sugar:**
GI: Low to medium
GL: Low
Sugar: 4g per teaspoon
Carbohydrates: 4g per teaspoon
Calories: 15 per teaspoon

**Yacon Syrup:**
GI: Low
GL: Low
Sugar: 6g per tablespoon
Carbohydrates: 6g per tablespoon
Calories: 20 per tablespoon

**Date Sugar:**
GI: Low to medium
GL: Low
Sugar: 4g per teaspoon
Carbohydrates: 4g per teaspoon
Calories: 15 per teaspoon

**Lucuma Powder:**
GI: Low
GL: Low
Sugar: 2g per tablespoon
Carbohydrates: 4g per tablespoon
Calories: 20 per tablespoon

**Chicory Root Fiber (Inulin):**
GI: Low
GL: Low
Sugar: 0g per teaspoon
Carbohydrates: 1g per teaspoon
Calories: 1.5 per gram

**Allulose:**
GI: Low
GL: Low
Sugar: 0g per teaspoon
Carbohydrates: 5g per teaspoon
Calories: 0.4 per gram

**Tagatose:**
GI: Low
GL: Low
Sugar: 0g per teaspoon
Carbohydrates: 5g per teaspoon
Calories: 1.5 per gram

**Inulin Syrup:**
GI: Low
GL: Low
Sugar: 5g per tablespoon
Carbohydrates: 5g per tablespoon
Calories: 20 per tablespoon

**Sorbitol (Sugar Alcohol):**
GI: Low
GL: Low
Sugar: 0g per teaspoon
Carbohydrates: 4g per teaspoon
Calories: 2.6 per gram

**Maltitol (Sugar Alcohol):**
GI: Low
GL: Low
Sugar: 0g per teaspoon
Carbohydrates: 4g per teaspoon
Calories: 2.1 per gram

**Lakanto (Monk Fruit and Erythritol Blend):**
GI: Low
GL: Low
Sugar: 0g per teaspoon
Carbohydrates: 4g per teaspoon
Calories: 0.2 per gram

**Sesame Date Balls (Homemade):**
GI: Low to medium
GL: Low
Sugar: Varies based on recipe
Carbohydrates: Varies based on recipe
Calories: Varies based on recipe

**Cacao Nibs (Unsweetened):**
GI: Low
GL: Low
Sugar: 0g per tablespoon
Carbohydrates: 4g per tablespoon
Calories: 50 per tablespoon

**Almond Butter (Unsweetened):**
GI: Low
GL: Low
Sugar: 0g per tablespoon
Carbohydrates: 3g per tablespoon
Calories: 98 per tablespoon

**Cashew Butter (Unsweetened):**
GI: Low
GL: Low
Sugar: 1g per tablespoon
Carbohydrates: 7g per tablespoon
Calories: 94 per tablespoon

**Pumpkin Puree (Unsweetened):**
GI: Low
GL: Low
Sugar: 1g per tablespoon
Carbohydrates: 3g per tablespoon
Calories: 15 per tablespoon

**Chia Seed Jam (Homemade):**
GI: Low
GL: Low
Sugar: Varies based on recipe
Carbohydrates: Varies based on recipe
Calories: Varies based on recipe

**Cottage Cheese with Berries:**
GI: Low
GL: Low
Sugar: 4g per half cup
Carbohydrates: 6g per half cup
Calories: 90 per half cup

**Greek Yogurt with Cinnamon:**
GI: Low
GL: Low
Sugar: 6g per half cup
Carbohydrates: 8g per half cup
Calories: 100 per half cup

***Avocado Chocolate Mousse (Homemade):***
GI: Low
GL: Low
Sugar: Varies based on recipe
Carbohydrates: Varies based on recipe
Calories: Varies based on recipe

**Homemade Berry Sorbet:**
GI: Low
GL: Low
Sugar: Varies based on recipe
Carbohydrates: Varies based on recipe
Calories: Varies based on recipe

**Homemade Applesauce (Unsweetened):**
GI: Low to medium
GL: Low
Sugar: Varies based on recipe
Carbohydrates: Varies based on recipe
Calories: Varies based on recipe

**Peach Slices (Fresh):**
GI: Low
GL: Low
Sugar: 8g per medium peach
Carbohydrates: 20g per medium peach
Calories: 60 per medium peach

**Pear Halves (Fresh):**
GI: Low
GL: Low
Sugar: 10g per medium pear
Carbohydrates: 27g per medium pear
Calories: 100 per medium pear

**Homemade Lemon Sorbet:**
GI: Low
GL: Low
Sugar: Varies based on recipe
Carbohydrates: Varies based on recipe
Calories: Varies based on recipe


## Snacks

**Greek Yogurt with Berries:**
GI: Low
GL: Low
Sugar: 8g per 6-ounce serving
Carbohydrates: 20g per 6-ounce serving
Calories: 150 per 6-ounce serving

**Hummus with Carrot Sticks:**
GI: Low
GL: Low
Sugar: 0.5g per 2 tablespoons
Carbohydrates: 6g per 2 tablespoons
Calories: 70 per 2 tablespoons

**Almonds (Raw):**
GI: Low
GL: Low
Sugar: 0.2g per ounce
Carbohydrates: 6g per ounce
Calories: 160 per ounce

**String Cheese:**
GI: Low
GL: Low
Sugar: 0.7g per stick
Carbohydrates: 1g per stick
Calories: 80 per stick

**Hard-Boiled Eggs:**
GI: Low
GL: Low
Sugar: 0g per egg
Carbohydrates: 0.6g per egg
Calories: 68 per egg

**Cherry Tomatoes with Mozzarella Balls:**
GI: Low
GL: Low
Sugar: 2g per cup
Carbohydrates: 4g per cup
Calories: 80 per cup

**Cottage Cheese with Pineapple:**
GI: Low
GL: Low
Sugar: 10g per 1/2 cup
Carbohydrates: 15g per 1/2 cup
Calories: 120 per 1/2 cup

**Avocado Slices with Sea Salt:**
GI: Low
GL: Low
Sugar: 0.2g per ounce
Carbohydrates: 3.4g per ounce
Calories: 45 per ounce

**Cucumber Slices with Tzatziki:**
GI: Low
GL: Low
Sugar: 1.5g per 1/2 cup
Carbohydrates: 3g per 1/2 cup
Calories: 50 per 1/2 cup

**Edamame (Steamed):**
GI: Low
GL: Low
Sugar: 2g per cup
Carbohydrates: 8g per cup
Calories: 94 per cup

**Peanut Butter (Natural) with Celery Sticks:**
GI: Low
GL: Low
Sugar: 1g per tablespoon
Carbohydrates: 6g per tablespoon
Calories: 94 per tablespoon

**Berries (Mixed):**
GI: Low
GL: Low
Sugar: 9g per cup
Carbohydrates: 23g per cup
Calories: 84 per cup

**Air-Popped Popcorn:**
GI: Low
GL: Low
Sugar: 0g per 3 cups
Carbohydrates: 15g per 3 cups
Calories: 93 per 3 cups

**Dark Chocolate (70% Cocoa):**
GI: Low to medium
GL: Low
Sugar: 6g per ounce
Carbohydrates: 15g per ounce
Calories: 170 per ounce

**Walnuts:**

GI: Low

GL: Low

Sugar: 0.7g per ounce

Carbohydrates: 3.9g per ounce

Calories: 185 per ounce

**Yogurt-Covered Strawberries:**

GI: Low to medium

GL: Low

Sugar: 17g per 1/2 cup

Carbohydrates: 40g per 1/2 cup

Calories: 180 per 1/2 cup

**Apple Slices with Almond Butter:**

GI: Low to medium

GL: Low

Sugar: 9g per medium apple

Carbohydrates: 25g per medium apple

Calories: 95 per medium apple

**Roasted Chickpeas:**

GI: Low

GL: Low

Sugar: 3g per 1/2 cup

Carbohydrates: 28g per 1/2 cup

Calories: 134 per 1/2 cup

**Dried Seaweed Snacks:**
GI: Low
GL: Low
Sugar: 0g per sheet
Carbohydrates: 1g per sheet
Calories: 5 per sheet

**Rice Cakes with Cream Cheese and Sliced Strawberries:**
GI: Low to medium
GL: Low
Sugar: 3g per rice cake
Carbohydrates: 22g per rice cake
Calories: 150 per rice cake

**Trail Mix (Nuts and Dried Berries):**
GI: Low
GL: Low
Sugar: 10g per 1/4 cup
Carbohydrates: 15g per 1/4 cup
Calories: 160 per 1/4 cup

**Cheese and Whole Grain Crackers:**
GI: Low
GL: Low
Sugar: 0.5g per serving
Carbohydrates: 15g per serving
Calories: 180 per serving

**Chia Seed Pudding:**
GI: Low
GL: Low
Sugar: 10g per cup
Carbohydrates: 33g per cup
Calories: 180 per cup

**Sliced Bell Peppers with Guacamole:**
GI: Low
GL: Low
Sugar: 2.5g per cup
Carbohydrates: 7g per cup
Calories: 100 per cup

**Frozen Grapes:**
GI: Low to medium
GL: Low
Sugar: 23g per cup
Carbohydrates: 23g per cup
Calories: 104 per cup

**Baked Kale Chips:**
GI: Low
GL: Low
Sugar: 0g per cup
Carbohydrates: 6g per cup
Calories: 50 per cup

**Jerky (Beef or Turkey):**
GI: Low
GL: Low
Sugar: 1g per ounce
Carbohydrates: 1g per ounce
Calories: 80 per ounce

**Pistachios (In Shell):**
GI: Low
GL: Low
Sugar: 2g per ounce
Carbohydrates: 8g per ounce
Calories: 160 per ounce

**Crudités with Yogurt-Based Dip:**
GI: Low
GL: Low
Sugar: 1g per cup
Carbohydrates: 5g per cup
Calories: 30 per cup

**Protein Bars (Low Sugar):**
GI: Low to medium
GL: Low
Sugar: 3g per bar
Carbohydrates: 20g per bar
Calories: 200 per bar

**Chicken Breast (Grilled):**
Protein: 31g per 3 ounces
Carbohydrates: 0g
Sugar: 0g
Calories: 165

**Salmon (Baked):**
Protein: 25g per 3 ounces
Carbohydrates: 0g
Sugar: 0g
Calories: 175

**Tofu (Firm):**
Protein: 10g per 1/2 cup
Carbohydrates: 2g
Sugar: 0g
Calories: 94

**Eggs (Hard-Boiled):**
Protein: 6g per egg
Carbohydrates: 1g
Sugar: 0g
Calories: 68

**Greek Yogurt (Plain, Non-fat):**
Protein: 15g per 6 ounces
Carbohydrates: 9g
Sugar: 6g
Calories: 100

**Black Beans (Cooked):**
Protein: 15g per 1 cup
Carbohydrates: 41g
Sugar: 0g
Calories: 227

**Cottage Cheese (Low-fat):**
Protein: 28g per 1 cup
Carbohydrates: 6g
Sugar: 5g
Calories: 206

**Turkey Breast (Roasted):**
Protein: 24g per 3 ounces
Carbohydrates: 0g
Sugar: 0g
Calories: 135

**Lentils (Cooked):**
Protein: 18g per 1 cup
Carbohydrates: 40g
Sugar: 4g
Calories: 230

**Shrimp (Grilled):**
Protein: 20g per 3 ounces
Carbohydrates: 0g
Sugar: 0g
Calories: 84

**Quinoa (Cooked):**
Protein: 8g per 1 cup
Carbohydrates: 39g
Sugar: 1g
Calories: 222

**Chickpeas (Cooked):**
Protein: 15g per 1 cup
Carbohydrates: 45g
Sugar: 8g
Calories: 269

**Pork Tenderloin (Grilled):**
Protein: 22g per 3 ounces
Carbohydrates: 0g
Sugar: 0g
Calories: 122

**Almonds (Roasted):**
Protein: 6g per 1 ounce
Carbohydrates: 6g
Sugar: 1g
Calories: 160

**Soy Milk (Unsweetened):**
Protein: 8g per 1 cup
Carbohydrates: 1g
Sugar: 0g
Calories: 80

**Beef (Grass-fed, Sirloin):**
Protein: 23g per 3 ounces
Carbohydrates: 0g
Sugar: 0g
Calories: 140

**Canned Tuna (in Water):**
Protein: 20g per 3 ounces
Carbohydrates: 0g
Sugar: 0g
Calories: 100

**Milk (Whole):**
Protein: 8g per 1 cup
Carbohydrates: 12g
Sugar: 12g
Calories: 150

**Walnuts:**
Protein: 4g per 1 ounce
Carbohydrates: 4g
Sugar: 1g
Calories: 185

**Cauliflower (Roasted):**
Protein: 3g per 1 cup
Carbohydrates: 5g
Sugar: 2g
Calories: 28

**Canned Chicken Breast (in Water):**
Protein: 22g per 3 ounces
Carbohydrates: 0g
Sugar: 0g
Calories: 98

**Yogurt (Whole Milk):**
Protein: 8g per 6 ounces
Carbohydrates: 8g
Sugar: 8g
Calories: 150

**Brazil Nuts:**
Protein: 4g per 1 ounce
Carbohydrates: 3g
Sugar: 1g
Calories: 190

**Edamame (Boiled):**
Protein: 17g per 1 cup
Carbohydrates: 16g
Sugar: 3g
Calories: 189

**Canned Salmon (Pink, Drained):**
Protein: 21g per 3 ounces
Carbohydrates: 0g
Sugar: 0g
Calories: 118

**Cheese (Cheddar):**
Protein: 7g per 1 ounce
Carbohydrates: 0g
Sugar: 0g
Calories: 115

**Peanut Butter (Natural):**
Protein: 7g per 2 tablespoons
Carbohydrates: 6g
Sugar: 1g
Calories: 180

**Spinach (Boiled):**
Protein: 6g per 1 cup
Carbohydrates: 6g
Sugar: 1g
Calories: 41

**Cheese (Mozzarella, Part-Skim):**
Protein: 9g per 1 ounce
Carbohydrates: 1g
Sugar: 0g
Calories: 72

**Pistachios (Roasted):**
Protein: 6g per 1 ounce
Carbohydrates: 8g
Sugar: 2g
Calories: 160

**Cheddar Cheese (Sharp):**
Carbohydrates: 0.4g per 1 ounce
Sugar: 0.1g
Calories: 113

**Mozzarella Cheese (Part-Skim):**
Carbohydrates: 1.6g per 1 ounce
Sugar: 0.6g
Calories: 72

**Feta Cheese (Reduced-Fat):**
Carbohydrates: 1g per 1 ounce
Sugar: 1g
Calories: 40

**Swiss Cheese:**
Carbohydrates: 1.5g per 1 ounce
Sugar: 0.1g
Calories: 111

**Blue Cheese:**
Carbohydrates: 0.7g per 1 ounce
Sugar: 0.2g
Calories: 100

**Goat Cheese (Soft):**
Carbohydrates: 0.6g per 1 ounce
Sugar: 0g
Calories: 76

**Parmesan Cheese (Grated):**
Carbohydrates: 0.9g per 1 tablespoon
Sugar: 0g
Calories: 22

**Cream Cheese (Reduced-Fat):**
Carbohydrates: 1.5g per 1 tablespoon
Sugar: 1g
Calories: 30

**Provolone Cheese:**
Carbohydrates: 0.6g per 1 ounce
Sugar: 0.1g
Calories: 98

**Cottage Cheese (Low-Fat):**
Carbohydrates: 6g per 1/2 cup
Sugar: 3g
Calories: 81

**Colby Cheese:**
Carbohydrates: 0.7g per 1 ounce
Sugar: 0.1g
Calories: 110

**Havarti Cheese:**
Carbohydrates: 0.1g per 1 ounce
Sugar: 0.1g
Calories: 110

**Monterey Jack Cheese:**
Carbohydrates: 0.4g per 1 ounce
Sugar: 0.1g
Calories: 104

**Ricotta Cheese (Part-Skim):**
Carbohydrates: 1g per 1 ounce
Sugar: 0g
Calories: 49

**Gouda Cheese**:
Carbohydrates: 0.6g per 1 ounce
Sugar: 0.1g
Calories: 110

**Brie Cheese:**
Carbohydrates: 0.1g per 1 ounce
Sugar: 0.1g
Calories: 94

**Pepper Jack Cheese:**
Carbohydrates: 0.1g per 1 ounce
Sugar: 0.1g
Calories: 100

**String Cheese (Part-Skim):**
Carbohydrates: 1g per 1 stick
Sugar: 0g
Calories: 80

**Limburger Cheese:**
Carbohydrates: 0.1g per 1 ounce
Sugar: 0.1g
Calories: 100

**Queso Fresco:**
Carbohydrates: 0.3g per 1 ounce
Sugar: 0.1g
Calories: 35

**Gruyère Cheese:**
Carbohydrates: 0.1g per 1 ounce
Sugar: 0.1g
Calories: 117

**Processed American Cheese (Singles):**
Carbohydrates: 2g per 1 slice
Sugar: 2g
Calories: 50

**Jarlsberg Cheese:**
Carbohydrates: 0.9g per 1 ounce
Sugar: 0.1g
Calories: 80

**Cotija Cheese:**
Carbohydrates: 0.1g per 1 tablespoon
Sugar: 0g
Calories: 20

**Muenster Cheese:**
Carbohydrates: 0.1g per 1 ounce
Sugar: 0.1g
Calories: 104

**Caciocavallo Cheese**:
Carbohydrates: 0.1g per 1 ounce
Sugar: 0.1g
Calories: 90

**Queso Blanco:**
Carbohydrates: 0.2g per 1 ounce
Sugar: 0.2g
Calories: 40

**Fontina Cheese:**
Carbohydrates: 0.1g per 1 ounce
Sugar: 0.1g
Calories: 110

**Emmental Cheese:**
Carbohydrates: 0.1g per 1 ounce
Sugar: 0.1g
Calories: 120

**Camembert Cheese:**
Carbohydrates: 0.1g per 1 ounce
Sugar: 0.1g
Calories: 85

## Spread and dips

**Hummus:**
Carbohydrates: 6g per 2 tablespoons
Sugar: 0g
Calories: 50

**Guacamole:**
Carbohydrates: 2g per 2 tablespoons
Sugar: 0g
Calories: 45

**Salsa (Fresh):**
Carbohydrates: 4g per 1/4 cup
Sugar: 2g
Calories: 15

**Tzatziki:**
Carbohydrates: 3g per 2 tablespoons
Sugar: 2g
Calories: 30

**Pesto (Basil):**
Carbohydrates: 1g per tablespoon
Sugar: 0g
Calories: 80

**Greek Yogurt Dip (Garlic and Herb):**
Carbohydrates: 3g per 2 tablespoons
Sugar: 2g
Calories: 30


**Peanut Butter (Natural):**
Carbohydrates: 6g per 2 tablespoons
Sugar: 1g
Calories: 180


**Sour Cream (Reduced-Fat):**
Carbohydrates: 3g per 2 tablespoons
Sugar: 2g
Calories: 40


**Cottage Cheese Dip (Spinach and Artichoke):**
Carbohydrates: 4g per 2 tablespoons
Sugar: 1g
Calories: 40


**Olive Tapenade:**
Carbohydrates: 1g per tablespoon
Sugar: 0g
Calories: 45


**Almond Butter (Natural):**
Carbohydrates: 6g per 2 tablespoons
Sugar: 1g
Calories: 190

**Ricotta Cheese Spread:**
Carbohydrates: 1g per 2 tablespoons
Sugar: 0g
Calories: 50

**Tahini:**
Carbohydrates: 3g per 2 tablespoons
Sugar: 0g
Calories: 180

**Cream Cheese (Light):**
Carbohydrates: 2g per 2 tablespoons
Sugar: 1g
Calories: 70

**Baba Ganoush:**
Carbohydrates: 3g per 2 tablespoons
Sugar: 1g
Calories: 50

**Sunflower Seed Butter (Natural):**
Carbohydrates: 5g per 2 tablespoons
Sugar: 1g
Calories: 190

**Yogurt Dip (Cucumber):**
Carbohydrates: 3g per 2 tablespoons
Sugar: 2g
Calories: 30

**Hot Sauce (Tabasco):**
Carbohydrates: 0g per teaspoon
Sugar: 0g
Calories: 0

**Artichoke Dip (Light):**
Carbohydrates: 2g per 2 tablespoons
Sugar: 0g
Calories: 30

**Chia Seed Jam (Strawberry):**
Carbohydrates: 5g per tablespoon
Sugar: 2g
Calories: 30

**Walnut Butter (Natural):**
Carbohydrates: 4g per 2 tablespoons
Sugar: 0g
Calories: 200

**Greek Yogurt Dip (Cilantro Lime):**
Carbohydrates: 3g per 2 tablespoons
Sugar: 2g
Calories: 30

**Honey Mustard Dip (Dijon):**
Carbohydrates: 3g per 2 tablespoons
Sugar: 2g
Calories: 60

**Chutney (Mango):**
Carbohydrates: 5g per 2 tablespoons
Sugar: 4g
Calories: 30

**Creamy Avocado Dressing:**
Carbohydrates: 2g per 2 tablespoons
Sugar: 0g
Calories: 50

**Peanut Sauce:**
Carbohydrates: 5g per 2 tablespoons
Sugar: 3g
Calories: 80

**Labneh (Strained Yogurt):**
Carbohydrates: 4g per 2 tablespoons
Sugar: 2g
Calories: 60

**Pumpkin Seed Butter (Natural):**
Carbohydrates: 6g per 2 tablespoons
Sugar: 1g
Calories: 180

**Soy Sauce (Low-Sodium):**
Carbohydrates: 1g per tablespoon
Sugar: 0g
Calories: 8

**Taramasalata (Fish Roe Spread):**
Carbohydrates: 2g per 2 tablespoons
Sugar: 0g
Calories: 80

## Dressings and marinades

**Balsamic Vinaigrette:**
Carbohydrates: 3g per 2 tablespoons
Sugar: 2g
Calories: 50

**Olive Oil and Lemon Dressing:**
Carbohydrates: 0g per 1 tablespoon
Sugar: 0g
Calories: 120

**Greek Yogurt Ranch Dressing:**
Carbohydrates: 2g per 2 tablespoons
Sugar: 1g
Calories: 50

**Sesame Ginger Marinade:**
Carbohydrates: 5g per 2 tablespoons
Sugar: 3g
Calories: 30

**Avocado Lime Dressing:**
Carbohydrates: 2g per 2 tablespoons
Sugar: 1g
Calories: 60

**Miso Sesame Dressing:**

Carbohydrates: 4g per 2 tablespoons

Sugar: 2g

Calories: 45


**Cilantro Lime Marinade:**

Carbohydrates: 4g per 2 tablespoons

Sugar: 1g

Calories: 30


**Honey Mustard Dressing:**

Carbohydrates: 5g per 2 tablespoons

Sugar: 4g

Calories: 70


**Tahini Lemon Dressing**

Carbohydrates: 2g per 2 tablespoons

Sugar: 0g

Calories: 90


**Red Wine Vinaigrette:**

Carbohydrates: 2g per 2 tablespoons

Sugar: 1g

Calories: 50


**Cilantro Lime Vinaigrette:**

Carbohydrates: 3g per 2 tablespoons

Sugar: 1g

Calories: 40

**Asian Peanut Sauce:**
Carbohydrates: 5g per 2 tablespoons
Sugar: 3g
Calories: 70

**Lemon Herb Marinade:**
Carbohydrates: 4g per 2 tablespoons
Sugar: 1g
Calories: 30

**Garlic Dijon Dressing:**
Carbohydrates: 1g per 1 tablespoon
Sugar: 0g
Calories: 50

**Yogurt Cucumber Dill Dressing:**
Carbohydrates: 3g per 2 tablespoons
Sugar: 2g
Calories: 40

**Soy Ginger Marinade:**
Carbohydrates: 5g per 2 tablespoons
Sugar: 3g
Calories: 30

**Maple Mustard Vinaigrette:**
Carbohydrates: 5g per 2 tablespoons
Sugar: 4g
Calories: 70

**Cranberry Orange Dressing:**
Carbohydrates: 4g per 2 tablespoons
Sugar: 3g
Calories: 45

**Lemon Garlic Tahini Dressing:**
Carbohydrates: 3g per 2 tablespoons
Sugar: 0g
Calories: 80

**Cajun Spice Marinade:**
Carbohydrates: 3g per 2 tablespoons
Sugar: 1g
Calories: 30

**Tomato Basil Vinaigrette:**
Carbohydrates: 4g per 2 tablespoons
Sugar: 3g
Calories: 50

**Chipotle Lime Dressing:**
Carbohydrates: 3g per 2 tablespoons
Sugar: 2g
Calories: 60

**Sesame Soy Marinade:**
Carbohydrates: 5g per 2 tablespoons
Sugar: 2g
Calories: 30

**Raspberry Walnut Vinaigrette:**
Carbohydrates: 3g per 2 tablespoons
Sugar: 2g
Calories: 50

**Yogurt Mint Sauce:**
Carbohydrates: 4g per 2 tablespoons
Sugar: 3g
Calories: 40

**Cumin Lime Marinade:**
Carbohydrates: 4g per 2 tablespoons
Sugar: 1g
Calories: 30

**Dill Pickle Dressing:**
Carbohydrates: 2g per 2 tablespoons
Sugar: 1g
Calories: 40

**Champagne Vinaigrette:**
Carbohydrates: 3g per 2 tablespoons
Sugar: 2g
Calories: 50

**Cranberry Balsamic Glaze:**
Carbohydrates: 5g per 2 tablespoons
Sugar: 3g
Calories: 50

**Pomegranate Molasses Dressing:**
Carbohydrates: 4g per 2 tablespoons
Sugar: 3g
Calories: 60

## Baking and Cooking ingredients

**Almond Flour:**
Carbohydrates: 6g per 1/4 cup
Sugar: 0g
Calories: 160

**Coconut Flour:**
Carbohydrates: 16g per 1/4 cup
Sugar: 4g
Calories: 120

**Oat Flour:**
Carbohydrates: 18g per 1/4 cup
Sugar: 0g
Calories: 120

**Stevia (Powdered):**
Carbohydrates: 1g per teaspoon
Sugar: 0g
Calories: 0

**Erythritol:**
Carbohydrates: 4g per 1 teaspoon
Sugar: 0g
Calories: 0

**Flaxseed Meal:**
Carbohydrates: 4g per 2 tablespoons
Sugar: 0g
Calories: 60

**Chia Seeds:**
Carbohydrates: 5g per 2 tablespoons
Sugar: 0g
Calories: 70

**Psyllium Husk Powder:**
Carbohydrates: 8g per 1 tablespoon
Sugar: 0g
Calories: 30

**Xanthan Gum:**
Carbohydrates: 7g per 1 tablespoon
Sugar: 0g
Calories: 30

**Unsweetened Cocoa Powder:**
Carbohydrates: 3g per 1 tablespoon
Sugar: 0g
Calories: 12

**Vanilla Extract:**
Carbohydrates: 1g per 1 teaspoon
Sugar: 0g
Calories: 12

**Baking Powder:**
Carbohydrates: 1g per 1 teaspoon
Sugar: 0g
Calories: 0

**Baking Soda:**
Carbohydrates: 0g per 1/2 teaspoon
Sugar: 0g
Calories: 0

**Unsweetened Applesauce:**
Carbohydrates: 13g per 1/4 cup
Sugar: 10g
Calories: 20

**Greek Yogurt (Plain, Unsweetened):**
Carbohydrates: 4g per 2 tablespoons
Sugar: 0g
Calories: 20

**Coconut Oil:**
Carbohydrates: 0g per 1 tablespoon
Sugar: 0g
Calories: 120

**Olive Oil:**
Carbohydrates: 0g per 1 tablespoon
Sugar: 0g
Calories: 120

**Butter (Unsalted):**
Carbohydrates: 0g per 1 tablespoon
Sugar: 0g
Calories: 100

**Eggs:**
Carbohydrates: 1g per large egg
Sugar: 0g
Calories: 70

**Yogurt (Plain, Unsweetened):**
Carbohydrates: 5g per 1/2 cup
Sugar: 4g
Calories: 50

**Almond Extract:**
Carbohydrates: 1g per 1 teaspoon
Sugar: 0g
Calories: 12

**Lemon Zest:**
Carbohydrates: 1g per 1 tablespoon
Sugar: 0g
Calories: 2

**Unsweetened Almond Milk:**
Carbohydrates: 1g per 1 cup
Sugar: 0g
Calories: 13

**Unsweetened Coconut Milk:**
Carbohydrates: 1g per 1 cup
Sugar: 0g
Calories: 50

**Coconut Extract:**
Carbohydrates: 1g per 1 teaspoon
Sugar: 0g
Calories: 12

**Almond Butter (Natural):**
Carbohydrates: 6g per 2 tablespoons
Sugar: 1g
Calories: 190

**Walnut Flour:**
Carbohydrates: 2g per 1/4 cup
Sugar: 0g
Calories: 150

**Hazelnut Flour:**
Carbohydrates: 3g per 1/4 cup
Sugar: 0g
Calories: 180

**Pumpkin Puree (Canned, Unsweetened):**
Carbohydrates: 8g per 1/2 cup
Sugar: 4g
Calories: 40

**Almond Meal:**
Carbohydrates: 6g per 1/4 cup
Sugar: 0g
Calories: 160

## Fat free and low dairy fat

**Fat-Free Greek Yogurt:**
Carbohydrates: 7g per 1/2 cup
Sugar: 6g
Calories: 60

**Low-Fat Cottage Cheese:**
Carbohydrates: 6g per 1/2 cup
Sugar: 3g
Calories: 90

**Skim Milk:**
Carbohydrates: 12g per 1 cup
Sugar: 12g
Calories: 80

**Fat-Free Ricotta Cheese:**
Carbohydrates: 7g per 1/2 cup
Sugar: 4g
Calories: 170

**Low-Fat Mozzarella Cheese:**
Carbohydrates: 1g per 1 ounce
Sugar: 0g
Calories: 50

**Fat-Free Sour Cream:**
Carbohydrates: 6g per 2 tablespoons
Sugar: 4g
Calories: 20

**Fat-Free Cream Cheese:**
Carbohydrates: 6g per 2 tablespoons
Sugar: 4g
Calories: 30

**Low-Fat Buttermilk:**
Carbohydrates: 12g per 1 cup
Sugar: 11g
Calories: 98

**Fat-Free Evaporated Milk:**
Carbohydrates: 20g per 1 cup
Sugar: 20g
Calories: 160

**Low-Fat Plain Yogurt:**
Carbohydrates: 17g per 1 cup
Sugar: 13g
Calories: 154

**Fat-Free Whipped Topping:**
Carbohydrates: 3g per 2 tablespoons
Sugar: 2g
Calories: 15

**Low-Fat Cheddar Cheese:**
Carbohydrates: 1g per 1 ounce
Sugar: 0g
Calories: 50

**Fat-Free Half-and-Half:**
Carbohydrates: 8g per 1 cup
Sugar: 6g
Calories: 120

**Low-Fat Swiss Cheese:**
Carbohydrates: 1g per 1 ounce
Sugar: 0g
Calories: 50

**Fat-Free American Cheese:**
Carbohydrates: 1g per 1 slice
Sugar: 0g
Calories: 30

**Low-Fat Plain Kefir:**
Carbohydrates: 12g per 1 cup
Sugar: 12g
Calories: 100

**Fat-Free Soy Milk:**
Carbohydrates: 8g per 1 cup
Sugar: 6g
Calories: 80

**Low-Fat Cottage Cheese (with fruit):**
Carbohydrates: 15g per 1/2 cup
Sugar: 11g
Calories: 100

**Fat-Free Yogurt (Flavored):**
Carbohydrates: 29g per 6 ounces
Sugar: 26g
Calories: 120

**Low-Fat String Cheese:**
Carbohydrates: 1g per 1 piece
Sugar: 0g
Calories: 50

**Fat-Free Chocolate Milk:**
Carbohydrates: 26g per 1 cup
Sugar: 24g
Calories: 150

**Low-Fat Plain Cream Cheese:**
Carbohydrates: 6g per 2 tablespoons
Sugar: 4g
Calories: 70

**Fat-Free Vanilla Yogurt:**
Carbohydrates: 38g per 8 ounces
Sugar: 37g
Calories: 180

**Low-Fat Colby Jack Cheese:**
Carbohydrates: 1g per 1 ounce
Sugar: 0g
Calories: 50

**Fat-Free Cottage Cheese (Small Curd):**
Carbohydrates: 6g per 1/2 cup
Sugar: 4g
Calories: 70

**Low-Fat Blue Cheese:**
Carbohydrates: 1g per 1 ounce
Sugar: 0g
Calories: 50

**Fat-Free Feta Cheese:**
Carbohydrates: 1g per 1 ounce
Sugar: 0g
Calories: 35

**Low-Fat Gouda Cheese:**
Carbohydrates: 1g per 1 ounce
Sugar: 0g
Calories: 50

**Fat-Free Irish Creamer:**
Carbohydrates: 9g per 1 cup
Sugar: 9g
Calories: 80

**Low-Fat Muenster Cheese:**
Carbohydrates: 1g per 1 ounce
Sugar: 0g
Calories: 50

## Fermented foods

**Sauerkraut:**
Carbohydrates: 2g per 1/2 cup
Sugar: 1g
Calories: 15

**Kimchi:**
Carbohydrates: 5g per 1/2 cup
Sugar: 2g
Calories: 22

**Miso Paste:**
Carbohydrates: 7g per tablespoon
Sugar: 2g
Calories: 34

**Tempeh:**
Carbohydrates: 9g per 3 ounces
Sugar: 0g
Calories: 160

**Natto:**
Carbohydrates: 11g per 1/2 cup
Sugar: 0g
Calories: 180

**Pickles (fermented without sugar):**
Carbohydrates: 1g per medium pickle
Sugar: 0g
Calories: 5

**Yogurt (Plain, Unsweetened):**
Carbohydrates: 11g per 1 cup
Sugar: 5g
Calories: 120

**Kombucha (Unsweetened):**
Carbohydrates: 2g per 8 ounces
Sugar: 0g
Calories: 30

**Sourdough Bread (Whole Grain):**
Carbohydrates: 15g per slice
Sugar: 0g
Calories: 80

**Fermented Pickled Radishes:**
Carbohydrates: 3g per 1/2 cup
Sugar: 0g
Calories: 15

**Fermented Garlic Dill Green Beans:**

Carbohydrates: 2g per 1/2 cup

Sugar: 0g

Calories: 15

**Fermented Carrots:**

Carbohydrates: 3g per 1/2 cup

Sugar: 0g

Calories: 15

**Fermented Beet Kvass:**

Carbohydrates: 2g per 1/2 cup

Sugar: 0g

Calories: 10

**Fermented Cabbage Juice:**

Carbohydrates: 2g per 1/2 cup

Sugar: 1g

Calories: 10

**Fermented Sweet Potato:**

Carbohydrates: 22g per 1 cup

Sugar: 5g

Calories: 112

**Fermented Tomato Salsa:**

Carbohydrates: 4g per 1/2 cup

Sugar: 2g

Calories: 20

**Fermented Bell Pepper Relish:**
Carbohydrates: 4g per 1/2 cup
Sugar: 2g
Calories: 20


**Fermented Cauliflower:**
Carbohydrates: 3g per 1/2 cup
Sugar: 1g
Calories: 15


**Fermented Eggplant:**
Carbohydrates: 5g per 1/2 cup
Sugar: 1g
Calories: 25


**Fermented Jalapenos:**
Carbohydrates: 3g per 1/2 cup
Sugar: 1g
Calories: 15


**Fermented Cucumber Salad:**
Carbohydrates: 2g per 1/2 cup
Sugar: 1g
Calories: 10


**Fermented Green Onion Kimchi:**
Carbohydrates: 4g per 1/2 cup
Sugar: 2g
Calories: 20

**Fermented Lemon Ginger Tea:**
Carbohydrates: 3g per 8 ounces
Sugar: 0g
Calories: 15

**Fermented Mango Chutney:**
Carbohydrates: 5g per 1/2 cup
Sugar: 3g
Calories: 25

**Fermented Pineapple Salsa:**
Carbohydrates: 5g per 1/2 cup
Sugar: 3g
Calories: 25

**Fermented Raspberry Vinegar:**
Carbohydrates: 4g per 1 tablespoon
Sugar: 3g
Calories: 20

**Fermented Watermelon Rind:**
Carbohydrates: 4g per 1/2 cup
Sugar: 2g
Calories: 20

**Fermented Zucchini Pickles:**
Carbohydrates: 2g per 1/2 cup
Sugar: 1g
Calories: 10

**Fermented Coconut Yogurt (Unsweetened):**
Carbohydrates: 7g per 1/2 cup
Sugar: 0g
Calories: 90

**Fermented Butternut Squash:**
Carbohydrates: 12g per 1 cup
Sugar: 0g
Calories: 50

Dietary Recommendations and Comprehensive Meal
Planning Tips for Glycemic Index

Embarking on a journey to incorporate the principles of the Glycemic Index (GI) into your dietary habits is a commendable step towards achieving optimal health. To make this transition seamless and effective, consider the following dietary recommendations and meal planning tips:

## Dietary Recommendations:

### Embrace Whole Foods:

Prioritize whole, minimally processed foods. These include fruits, vegetables, whole grains, lean proteins, and legumes. Whole foods generally have a lower GI, promoting stable blood sugar levels.

### Balanced Macronutrients:

Aim for balanced meals that include a mix of carbohydrates, proteins, and healthy fats. This combination helps slow down the digestion and absorption of carbohydrates, mitigating spikes in blood sugar.

### Favor Low-Glycemic Carbohydrates:

Choose carbohydrates with a low GI, such as sweet potatoes, quinoa, and whole grain options. These release glucose gradually, providing sustained energy and promoting satiety.

### Include Fiber-Rich Foods:
Fiber-rich foods like vegetables, fruits, and whole grains not only contribute to a lower GI but also aid in digestion and contribute to a feeling of fullness.

### Mindful Portion Control:
Be conscious of portion sizes. Even low-GI foods can impact blood sugar levels if consumed excessively. Consider using smaller plates to help with portion control.

### Lean Protein Choices:
Incorporate lean protein sources like poultry, fish, tofu, and legumes. Protein-rich foods contribute to a feeling of fullness and help regulate blood sugar.

### Healthy Fats:
Include sources of healthy fats, such as avocados, nuts, and olive oil. These fats contribute to satiety and add flavor to meals without significantly impacting the GI.

### Hydration is Key:
Stay adequately hydrated. Water is essential for various bodily functions, including digestion. Consider water-rich foods like fruits and vegetables.

**Limit Processed and Refined Foods:**
Minimize the intake of highly processed and refined foods, as they often have a higher GI. Opt for whole, nutrient-dense alternatives.

## Comprehensive Meal Planning Tips

**Create a Balanced Plate:**
Structure meals to include a variety of colorful vegetables, lean proteins, whole grains, and healthy fats. This ensures a balance of nutrients and flavors.

**Prep Ahead for Convenience:**
Plan and prepare meals in advance, especially if time is a constraint. This reduces the likelihood of opting for convenient but less nutritious choices.

**Diversify Your Menu:**
Explore a diverse range of low-GI foods to keep meals interesting. Experiment with different grains, vegetables, and proteins to discover new favorites.

**Snack Smartly:**
Choose snacks with a combination of protein and fiber to maintain energy levels between meals. Greek yogurt with berries or vegetable sticks with hummus are excellent options.

**Read Food Labels:**
Familiarize yourself with food labels to identify hidden sugars and processed ingredients. Opt for products with lower GI values.

**Mindful Eating Practices:**
Practice mindful eating by savoring each bite, eating slowly, and paying attention to hunger and fullness cues. This promotes a healthier relationship with food.

**Include a Variety of Cooking Methods:**
Experiment with different cooking methods—grilling, roasting, steaming—to enhance flavors without compromising the nutritional integrity of the food.

**Consult a Registered Dietitian:**
Consider consulting a registered dietitian for personalized guidance. They can help tailor dietary recommendations based on individual health goals, preferences, and medical conditions.

## Low-GI Breakfast

**Oatmeal (Steel-Cut):**
Glycemic Index: 42
Glycemic Load: 13
Carbohydrates: 27g per 1/2 cup (uncooked)
Sugar: 1g
Calories: 150

**Greek Yogurt (Plain, Unsweetened):**
Glycemic Index: 11
Glycemic Load: 3
Carbohydrates: 6g per 100g
Sugar: 4g
Calories: 59

**Egg Omelette with Vegetables:**
Glycemic Index: N/A
Glycemic Load: N/A
Carbohydrates: 2g per egg
Sugar: 1g
Calories: 94

**Chia Seed Pudding:**
Glycemic Index: 1
Glycemic Load: 0
Carbohydrates: 12g per 2 tablespoons

Sugar: 0g
Calories: 90

**Whole Grain Toast with Avocado:**
Glycemic Index: 50
Glycemic Load: 9
Carbohydrates: 15g per slice
Sugar: 1g
Calories: 80

**Berries (Mixed):**
Glycemic Index: 40
Glycemic Load: 5
Carbohydrates: 11g per 1/2 cup
Sugar: 6g
Calories: 29

**Cottage Cheese (Low-Fat):**
Glycemic Index: 10
Glycemic Load: 3
Carbohydrates: 6g per 100g
Sugar: 3g
Calories: 72

**Smoothie with Green Leafy Vegetables and Berries:**
Glycemic Index: N/A
Glycemic Load: N/A
Carbohydrates: 20g per cup
Sugar: 10g
Calories: 80

**Almond Butter on Whole Grain Bread:**
Glycemic Index: 30
Glycemic Load: 5
Carbohydrates: 15g per slice
Sugar: 1g
Calories: 94

**Quinoa Porridge:**
Glycemic Index: 53
Glycemic Load: 13
Carbohydrates: 21g per 1/2 cup (cooked)
Sugar: 0g
Calories: 111

**Walnut and Banana Smoothie:**
Glycemic Index: N/A
Glycemic Load: N/A
Carbohydrates: 30g per cup
Sugar: 15g
Calories: 200

**Cauliflower Hash Browns:**
Glycemic Index: N/A
Glycemic Load: N/A
Carbohydrates: 4g per 1/2 cup
Sugar: 2g
Calories: 50

**Salmon and Avocado Wrap:**
Glycemic Index: N/A
Glycemic Load: N/A
Carbohydrates: 22g per wrap
Sugar: 2g
Calories: 300

**Rye Bread with Smoked Salmon:**
Glycemic Index: 45
Glycemic Load: 6
Carbohydrates: 15g per slice
Sugar: 0g
Calories: 83

**Mushroom and Spinach Frittata:**
Glycemic Index: N/A
Glycemic Load: N/A
Carbohydrates: 5g per serving
Sugar: 2g
Calories: 150

**Apple Slices with Almond Butter:**
Glycemic Index: 25
Glycemic Load: 3
Carbohydrates: 19g per medium apple
Sugar: 14g
Calories: 95

**Brown Rice Cake with Hummus:**
Glycemic Index: 50
Glycemic Load: 8
Carbohydrates: 15g per cake
Sugar: 0g
Calories: 70

**Cinnamon and Vanilla Protein Pancakes:**
Glycemic Index: 45
Glycemic Load: 10
Carbohydrates: 20g per 2 pancakes
Sugar: 3g
Calories: 180

**Sardines on Whole Grain Crackers:**
Glycemic Index: 15
Glycemic Load: 1
Carbohydrates: 10g per 5 crackers
Sugar: 0g
Calories: 100

**Sweet Potato Hash with Poached Eggs:**
Glycemic Index: 50
Glycemic Load: 10
Carbohydrates: 20g per serving
Sugar: 2g
Calories: 250

**Green Tea:**
Glycemic Index: N/A
Glycemic Load: N/A
Carbohydrates: 0g per cup
Sugar: 0g
Calories: 0

**Cottage Cheese and Pineapple Bowl:**
Glycemic Index: 65 (for pineapple)
Glycemic Load: 10 (for pineapple)
Carbohydrates: 15g per 1/2 cup (cottage cheese)
Sugar: 8g
Calories: 104

**Smoked Turkey and Cheese Roll-Ups:**
Glycemic Index: N/A
Glycemic Load: N/A
Carbohydrates: 2g per roll-up
Sugar: 0g
Calories: 50

**Soy Milk (Unsweetened):**
Glycemic Index: 44
Glycemic Load: 4
Carbohydrates: 4g per cup
Sugar: 1g
Calories: 40

**Peanut Butter Banana Toast:**
Glycemic Index: 41
Glycemic Load: 9
Carbohydrates: 30g per slice
Sugar: 10g
Calories: 200

**Cocoa Chia Seed Pudding:**
Glycemic Index: 1
Glycemic Load: 0
Carbohydrates: 12g per 2 tablespoons
Sugar: 0g
Calories: 90

**Salmon and Cream Cheese Bagel:**
Glycemic Index: 72 (for bagel)
Glycemic Load: 25 (for bagel)
Carbohydrates: 6g per 2 tablespoons (cream cheese)
Sugar: 2g
Calories: 350

**Blueberry Almond Smoothie:**
Glycemic Index: N/A
Glycemic Load: N/A
Carbohydrates: 20g per cup
Sugar: 10g
Calories: 150

**Sesame Seed Oat Bar:**
Glycemic Index: 50
Glycemic Load: 12
Carbohydrates: 30g per bar
Sugar: 8g
Calories: 200

**Shakshuka:**
Glycemic Index: N/A
Glycemic Load: N/A
Carbohydrates: 10g per serving
Sugar: 6g
Calories: 200

## Low-GI Lunch

**Grilled Chicken Salad:**
Glycemic Index: N/A
Glycemic Load: N/A
Carbohydrates: 5g per serving
Sugar: 2g
Calories: 250

**Quinoa and Black Bean Bowl:**
Glycemic Index: 53
Glycemic Load: 13
Carbohydrates: 30g per cup (cooked)
Sugar: 1g
Calories: 220

**Salmon and Avocado Wrap:**
Glycemic Index: N/A
Glycemic Load: N/A
Carbohydrates: 22g per wrap
Sugar: 2g
Calories: 300

**Lentil Soup:**
Glycemic Index: 29
Glycemic Load: 5
Carbohydrates: 20g per cup
Sugar: 2g
Calories: 200

**Vegetarian Stir-Fry with Tofu:**
Glycemic Index: N/A
Glycemic Load: N/A
Carbohydrates: 25g per serving
Sugar: 8g
Calories: 300

**Turkey and Vegetable Lettuce Wraps:**
Glycemic Index: N/A
Glycemic Load: N/A
Carbohydrates: 10g per serving
Sugar: 4g
Calories: 180

**Chickpea Salad with Feta:**
Glycemic Index: 28
Glycemic Load: 9
Carbohydrates: 30g per cup
Sugar: 4g
Calories: 200

**Brown Rice and Vegetable Sushi Rolls:**
Glycemic Index: 50
Glycemic Load: 15
Carbohydrates: 40g per 6 pieces
Sugar: 2g
Calories: 250

**Eggplant Parmesan:**
Glycemic Index: 15
Glycemic Load: 3
Carbohydrates: 15g per serving
Sugar: 6g
Calories: 220

**Cauliflower Rice Burrito Bowl:**
Glycemic Index: N/A
Glycemic Load: N/A
Carbohydrates: 20g per serving
Sugar: 5g
Calories: 280

**Shrimp and Asparagus Stir-Fry:**
Glycemic Index: N/A
Glycemic Load: N/A
Carbohydrates: 15g per serving
Sugar: 4g
Calories: 230

**Mushroom and Spinach Quiche:**
Glycemic Index: N/A
Glycemic Load: N/A
Carbohydrates: 20g per slice
Sugar: 2g
Calories: 180

**Chickpea and Spinach Stew:**
Glycemic Index: 33
Glycemic Load: 8
Carbohydrates: 25g per cup
Sugar: 2g
Calories: 220

**Cabbage and Turkey Sauté:**
Glycemic Index: N/A
Glycemic Load: N/A
Carbohydrates: 15g per serving
Sugar: 5g
Calories: 180

**Whole Grain Wrap with Hummus and Veggies:**
Glycemic Index: 30
Glycemic Load: 10
Carbohydrates: 30g per wrap
Sugar: 4g
Calories: 250

**Salmon and Quinoa Stuffed Bell Peppers:**
Glycemic Index: N/A
Glycemic Load: N/A
Carbohydrates: 30g per serving
Sugar: 5g
Calories: 280

**Spinach and Feta Turkey Burger:**
Glycemic Index: N/A
Glycemic Load: N/A
Carbohydrates: 20g per burger
Sugar: 2g
Calories: 220

**Tuna and White Bean Salad:**
Glycemic Index: N/A
Glycemic Load: N/A
Carbohydrates: 15g per serving
Sugar: 1g
Calories: 180

**Sweet Potato and Black Bean Quesadilla:**
Glycemic Index: 44
Glycemic Load: 20
Carbohydrates: 45g per quesadilla
Sugar: 5g
Calories: 350

**Broccoli and Chicken Alfredo (with Whole Grain Pasta):**
Glycemic Index: 32
Glycemic Load: 15
Carbohydrates: 40g per serving
Sugar: 2g
Calories: 300

**Caprese Salad with Balsamic Glaze:**
Glycemic Index: N/A
Glycemic Load: N/A
Carbohydrates: 10g per serving
Sugar: 5g
Calories: 150

**Pesto Zucchini Noodles with Cherry Tomatoes:**
Glycemic Index: N/A
Glycemic Load: N/A
Carbohydrates: 15g per serving
Sugar: 4g
Calories: 180

**Stuffed Bell Peppers with Ground Turkey and Quinoa:**
Glycemic Index: N/A
Glycemic Load: N/A
Carbohydrates: 30g per serving
Sugar: 5g
Calories: 280

**Cauliflower and Broccoli Soup:**
Glycemic Index: 25
Glycemic Load: 5
Carbohydrates: 20g per cup
Sugar: 5g
Calories: 150

**Grilled Veggie and Chicken Kabobs:**
Glycemic Index: N/A
Glycemic Load: N/A
Carbohydrates: 15g per skewer
Sugar: 6g
Calories: 200

**Chia Seed and Berry Smoothie Bowl:**
Glycemic Index: 1
Glycemic Load: 0
Carbohydrates: 30g per bowl
Sugar: 10g
Calories: 220

**Egg Salad Lettuce Wraps:**
Glycemic Index: N/A
Glycemic Load: N/A
Carbohydrates: 10g per serving
Sugar: 2g
Calories: 120

**Mediterranean Chickpea Salad:**
Glycemic Index: 28
Glycemic Load: 7
Carbohydrates: 25g per cup
Sugar: 4g
Calories: 200

**Cajun Shrimp and Quinoa:**
Glycemic Index: N/A
Glycemic Load: N/A
Carbohydrates: 30g per serving
Sugar: 3g
Calories: 250

**Pumpkin and Lentil Curry:**
Glycemic Index: N/A
Glycemic Load: N/A
Carbohydrates: 35g per serving
Sugar: 5g
Calories: 300

Baked Salmon with Lemon and Herbs:
Glycemic Index: N/A
Glycemic Load: N/A
Carbohydrates: 0g
Sugar: 0g
Calories: 200 per 3-ounce serving

**Cauliflower and Broccoli Gratin:**
Glycemic Index: 25
Glycemic Load: 5
Carbohydrates: 15g per serving
Sugar: 5g
Calories: 180

**Grilled Chicken Breast with Asparagus:**
Glycemic Index: N/A
Glycemic Load: N/A
Carbohydrates: 0g
Sugar: 0g
Calories: 250 per 4-ounce serving

**Lentil and Vegetable Stew:**
Glycemic Index: 29
Glycemic Load: 5
Carbohydrates: 20g per cup
Sugar: 2g
Calories: 200

**Turkey and Spinach Stuffed Bell Peppers:**
Glycemic Index: N/A
Glycemic Load: N/A
Carbohydrates: 15g per pepper
Sugar: 5g
Calories: 250

**Shrimp and Vegetable Stir-Fry:**
Glycemic Index: N/A
Glycemic Load: N/A
Carbohydrates: 15g per serving
Sugar: 4g
Calories: 230

**Quinoa and Black Bean Casserole:**
Glycemic Index: 53
Glycemic Load: 13
Carbohydrates: 30g per cup (cooked)
Sugar: 1g
Calories: 220

**Grilled Eggplant and Zucchini Skewers:**
Glycemic Index: N/A
Glycemic Load: N/A
Carbohydrates: 10g per serving
Sugar: 3g
Calories: 180

**Mushroom and Spinach Stuffed Chicken Breast:**
Glycemic Index: N/A
Glycemic Load: N/A
Carbohydrates: 2g
Sugar: 0g
Calories: 200 per 4-ounce serving

**Chickpea and Vegetable Curry:**
Glycemic Index: 33
Glycemic Load: 8
Carbohydrates: 25g per cup
Sugar: 2g
Calories: 220

**Salmon and Quinoa Salad:**
Glycemic Index: N/A
Glycemic Load: N/A
Carbohydrates: 30g per serving
Sugar: 5g
Calories: 280

**Cabbage and Chicken Sauté:**
Glycemic Index: N/A
Glycemic Load: N/A
Carbohydrates: 10g per serving
Sugar: 4g
Calories: 200

**Grilled Portobello Mushrooms with Balsamic Glaze:**
Glycemic Index: N/A
Glycemic Load: N/A
Carbohydrates: 5g per serving
Sugar: 3g
Calories: 120

**Spaghetti Squash with Tomato Sauce and Turkey Meatballs:**
Glycemic Index: 32
Glycemic Load: 12
Carbohydrates: 30g per serving
Sugar: 8g
Calories: 250

**Chia Seed and Vegetable Stuffed Peppers:**
Glycemic Index: N/A
Glycemic Load: N/A
Carbohydrates: 20g per pepper
Sugar: 5g
Calories: 180

**Tofu and Broccoli Stir-Fry:**
Glycemic Index: N/A
Glycemic Load: N/A
Carbohydrates: 15g per serving
Sugar: 4g
Calories: 230

**Lemon Herb Grilled Chicken with Roasted Vegetables:**
Glycemic Index: N/A
Glycemic Load: N/A
Carbohydrates: 10g per serving
Sugar: 4g
Calories: 280

**Quinoa and Chickpea Pilaf:**
Glycemic Index: 53
Glycemic Load: 13
Carbohydrates: 30g per cup (cooked)
Sugar: 1g
Calories: 220

**Cauliflower and Spinach Curry:**
Glycemic Index: 32
Glycemic Load: 12
Carbohydrates: 25g per cup
Sugar: 2g
Calories: 200

**Turkey and Vegetable Skillet:**
Glycemic Index: N/A
Glycemic Load: N/A
Carbohydrates: 15g per serving
Sugar: 4g
Calories: 230

**Stuffed Acorn Squash with Quinoa and Cranberries:**
Glycemic Index: 65 (for cranberries)
Glycemic Load: 10 (for cranberries)
Carbohydrates: 30g per squash
Sugar: 5g
Calories: 280

**Egg Fried Cauliflower Rice:**
Glycemic Index: N/A
Glycemic Load: N/A
Carbohydrates: 10g per serving
Sugar: 3g
Calories: 150

**Baked Cod with Tomato and Olive Tapenade:**
Glycemic Index: N/A
Glycemic Load: N/A
Carbohydrates: 5g per serving
Sugar: 2g
Calories: 180

**Mushroom and Spinach Stuffed Bell Peppers:**
Glycemic Index: N/A
Glycemic Load: N/A
Carbohydrates: 15g per pepper
Sugar: 5g
Calories: 250

**Cajun Chicken and Vegetable Skewers:**
Glycemic Index: N/A
Glycemic Load: N/A
Carbohydrates: 10g per skewer
Sugar: 4g
Calories: 200

**Chickpea and Kale Stew:**
Glycemic Index: 33
Glycemic Load: 8
Carbohydrates: 25g per cup
Sugar: 2g
Calories: 220

**Turkey and Sweet Potato Chili:**
Glycemic Index: 54
Glycemic Load: 14
Carbohydrates: 30g per cup
Sugar: 5g
Calories: 250

**Cabbage Roll Casserole:**
Glycemic Index: N/A
Glycemic Load: N/A
Carbohydrates: 15g per serving
Sugar: 5g
Calories: 180

**Grilled Zucchini and Eggplant Lasagna:**
Glycemic Index: 30
Glycemic Load: 10
Carbohydrates: 20g per serving
Sugar: 8g
Calories: 250

**Chickpea and Spinach Coconut Curry:**
Glycemic Index: 33
Glycemic Load: 8
Carbohydrates: 25g per cup
Sugar: 2g
Calories: 220

## Low-GI Snack Ideas

**Greek Yogurt with Berries:**
Glycemic Index: N/A
Glycemic Load: N/A
Carbohydrates: 15g per serving
Sugar: 8g
Calories: 150

**Hummus and Vegetable Sticks:**
Glycemic Index: N/A
Glycemic Load: N/A
Carbohydrates: 10g per serving
Sugar: 2g
Calories: 120

**Almonds and Walnuts Mix:**
Glycemic Index: N/A
Glycemic Load: N/A
Carbohydrates: 5g per serving
Sugar: 1g
Calories: 180

**Hard-Boiled Eggs:**
Glycemic Index: N/A
Glycemic Load: N/A
Carbohydrates: 1g per egg
Sugar: 0g
Calories: 70

**Cherry Tomatoes with Mozzarella:**
Glycemic Index: 22
Glycemic Load: 6
Carbohydrates: 5g per serving
Sugar: 3g
Calories: 100

**Cottage Cheese with Pineapple**:
Glycemic Index: 46
Glycemic Load: 6
Carbohydrates: 15g per serving
Sugar: 10g
Calories: 120

**Celery Sticks with Peanut Butter:**
Glycemic Index: N/A
Glycemic Load: N/A
Carbohydrates: 8g per serving
Sugar: 3g
Calories: 150

**Sliced Cucumber with Tzatziki:**
Glycemic Index: N/A
Glycemic Load: N/A
Carbohydrates: 5g per serving
Sugar: 2g
Calories: 80

**Berries Smoothie with Protein Powder:**
Glycemic Index: N/A
Glycemic Load: N/A
Carbohydrates: 20g per serving
Sugar: 10g
Calories: 200

**Edamame Beans:**
Glycemic Index: 30
Glycemic Load: 6
Carbohydrates: 8g per serving
Sugar: 2g
Calories: 100

**Avocado Slices with Salt and Pepper:**
Glycemic Index: N/A
Glycemic Load: N/A
Carbohydrates: 5g per serving
Sugar: 0g
Calories: 80

**Roasted Chickpeas:**
Glycemic Index: 28
Glycemic Load: 9
Carbohydrates: 30g per cup
Sugar: 4g
Calories: 200

**Cheese and Whole Grain Crackers:**
Glycemic Index: N/A
Glycemic Load: N/A
Carbohydrates: 15g per serving
Sugar: 2g
Calories: 180

**Sliced Apple with Almond Butter:**
Glycemic Index: 36
Glycemic Load: 5
Carbohydrates: 20g per apple
Sugar: 15g
Calories: 150

**Carrot Sticks with Guacamole:**
Glycemic Index: N/A
Glycemic Load: N/A
Carbohydrates: 10g per serving
Sugar: 2g
Calories: 120

**Yogurt Parfait with Nuts and Berries:**
Glycemic Index: N/A
Glycemic Load: N/A
Carbohydrates: 20g per serving
Sugar: 10g
Calories: 180

**Chia Seed Pudding with Unsweetened Almond Milk:**
Glycemic Index: 1
Glycemic Load: 0
Carbohydrates: 15g per serving
Sugar: 0g
Calories: 120

**Green Tea and a Handful of Almonds:**
Glycemic Index: N/A
Glycemic Load: N/A
Carbohydrates: 5g per serving
Sugar: 1g
Calories: 100

**Pear Slices with Cottage Cheese:**
Glycemic Index: 38
Glycemic Load: 4
Carbohydrates: 15g per pear
Sugar: 10g
Calories: 120

**Trail Mix with Dried Berries and Nuts:**
Glycemic Index: N/A
Glycemic Load: N/A
Carbohydrates: 15g per serving
Sugar: 8g
Calories: 180

**Smoked Salmon Roll-Ups:**
Glycemic Index: N/A
Glycemic Load: N/A
Carbohydrates: 2g per serving
Sugar: 0g
Calories: 80

**Cinnamon Roasted Almonds:**
Glycemic Index: N/A
Glycemic Load: N/A
Carbohydrates: 8g per serving
Sugar: 2g
Calories: 120

**Whole Grain Rice Cake with Avocado:**
Glycemic Index: 70
Glycemic Load: 17
Carbohydrates: 15g per rice cake
Sugar: 0g
Calories: 80

**Caprese Skewers (Cherry Tomatoes, Mozzarella, Basil):**
Glycemic Index: N/A
Glycemic Load: N/A
Carbohydrates: 5g per serving
Sugar: 2g
Calories: 100

**Sliced Peaches with Cottage Cheese:**
Glycemic Index: 42
Glycemic Load: 5
Carbohydrates: 15g per peach
Sugar: 10g
Calories: 120

**Dill Pickles Wrapped in Turkey Slices:**
Glycemic Index: N/A
Glycemic Load: N/A
Carbohydrates: 2g per serving
Sugar: 0g
Calories: 50

**Ricotta and Berry Parfait:**
Glycemic Index: N/A
Glycemic Load: N/A
Carbohydrates: 20g per serving
Sugar: 10g
Calories: 180

**Stuffed Dates with Almond Butter:**
Glycemic Index: 42
Glycemic Load: 12
Carbohydrates: 15g per date
Sugar: 10g
Calories: 120

**Brussels Sprouts Chips**:
Glycemic Index: N/A
Glycemic Load: N/A
Carbohydrates: 10g per serving
Sugar: 2g
Calories: 120

**Yogurt-Covered Strawberries:**
Glycemic Index: 25
Glycemic Load: 3
Carbohydrates: 15g per serving
Sugar: 10g
Calories: 120

# 45 DAYS LOW GLYCEMIC INDEX DIET MEAL PLAN

## Day 1:

Quinoa Salad Bowl

**Ingredients:**

1 cup cooked quinoa

Mixed vegetables (tomatoes, cucumbers, bell peppers)

Feta cheese

Olive oil, lemon juice, salt, and pepper for dressing

**Preparation:**

Mix cooked quinoa with chopped vegetables.

Add crumbled feta cheese.

Drizzle with olive oil, lemon juice, salt, and pepper.

Prep Time: 15 minutes

GI Value: 53

GI Load: 13

Carbohydrates: 30g per serving

Sugar: 1g

Calories: 220

## Day 2:

Baked Salmon with Asparagus

Ingredients:

Salmon fillets

Asparagus spears

Olive oil, garlic, lemon, salt, and pepper for seasoning

**Preparation:**
Season salmon and asparagus with olive oil, garlic, lemon, salt, and pepper.
Bake until salmon is cooked through.
Prep Time: 25 minutes
GI Value: N/A
GI Load: N/A
Carbohydrates: 0g
Sugar: 0g
Calories: 250

## Day 3:

Lentil and Vegetable Stew
Ingredients:
1 cup lentils
Mixed vegetables (carrots, celery, onions)
Vegetable broth, garlic, cumin, coriander

**Preparation:**
Cook lentils and set aside.
Sauté vegetables in garlic, add cumin and coriander.
Mix in lentils and vegetable broth.
Prep Time: 30 minutes
GI Value: 29
GI Load: 5
Carbohydrates: 20g per serving
Sugar: 2g
Calories: 200

## Day 4:

Greek Chicken Salad
Ingredients:
Grilled chicken breast
Mixed greens, cherry tomatoes, cucumber
Feta cheese, olives

**Preparation:**
Grill chicken and slice into strips.
Combine with mixed greens, cherry tomatoes, cucumber, feta, and olives.
Prep Time: 20 minutes
GI Value: N/A
GI Load: N/A
Carbohydrates: 15g per serving
Sugar: 3g
Calories: 180

## Day 5:

Cauliflower Fried Rice
Ingredients:
Grated cauliflower
Mixed vegetables (peas, carrots, onions)
Egg, soy sauce, garlic, ginger

**Preparation:**
Sauté vegetables, garlic, and ginger.
Add grated cauliflower, scramble in the egg, and stir in soy sauce.

Prep Time: 25 minutes
GI Value: N/A
GI Load: N/A
Carbohydrates: 10g per serving
Sugar: 3g
Calories: 150

## Day 6:

Turkey and Spinach Stuffed Bell Peppers
Ingredients:
Ground turkey
Spinach, tomatoes, black beans
Taco seasoning, cheese

**Preparation:**
Cook turkey with taco seasoning.
Stuff bell peppers with turkey mixture, spinach, tomatoes,
and black beans.
Prep Time: 35 minutes
GI Value: N/A
GI Load: N/A
Carbohydrates: 15g per serving
Sugar: 5g
Calories: 250

Chia Seed Pudding with Berries
Ingredients:
Chia seeds
Almond milk
Mixed berries
Honey for sweetness

**Preparation:**
Mix chia seeds and almond milk, refrigerate overnight.
Top with mixed berries and a drizzle of honey.
Prep Time: 10 minutes (+overnight chilling)
GI Value: 1
GI Load: 0
Carbohydrates: 15g per serving
Sugar: 0g
Calories: 120


Caprese Zucchini Noodles
Ingredients:
Zucchini noodles
Cherry tomatoes, mozzarella
Fresh basil, balsamic glaze

**Preparation:**
Spiralize zucchini into noodles.
Mix with cherry tomatoes, mozzarella, and fresh basil.
Prep Time: 15 minutes

GI Value: N/A
GI Load: N/A
Carbohydrates: 10g per serving
Sugar: 4g
Calories: 180

## Day 9:

Chickpea and Vegetable Stir-Fry
Ingredients:
Chickpeas
Mixed vegetables (broccoli, bell peppers, snap peas)
Soy sauce, garlic, ginger

**Preparation:**
Sauté vegetables, garlic, and ginger.
Add chickpeas and soy sauce, stir-fry until cooked.
Prep Time: 20 minutes
GI Value: N/A
GI Load: N/A
Carbohydrates: 15g per serving
Sugar: 4g
Calories: 230

## Day 10:

Baked Cod with Lemon and Herbs
Ingredients:
Cod fillets
Lemon, garlic, parsley

**Preparation:**
Season cod with lemon, garlic, and parsley.
Bake until cod is flaky.
Prep Time: 20 minutes
GI Value: N/A
GI Load: N/A
Carbohydrates: 5g per serving
Sugar: 2g
Calories: 180

## Day 11:

Eggplant and Tomato Stacks
Ingredients:
Eggplant slices
Tomato slices, mozzarella
Fresh basil, balsamic glaze

**Preparation:**
Grill eggplant slices.
Stack with tomato, mozzarella, and fresh basil. Drizzle with balsamic glaze.
Prep Time: 25 minutes
GI Value: N/A
GI Load: N/A
Carbohydrates: 15g per serving
Sugar: 5g
Calories: 200

Day 12:

Lentil and Spinach Salad
Ingredients:
Cooked lentils
Fresh spinach, cherry tomatoes
Feta cheese, balsamic vinaigrette

**Preparation:**
Toss lentils with fresh spinach and cherry tomatoes.
Top with crumbled feta and drizzle with balsamic vinaigrette.
Prep Time: 15 minutes
GI Value: 29
GI Load: 5
Carbohydrates: 20g per serving
Sugar: 2g
Calories: 220

Day 13:

Grilled Chicken and Vegetable Skewers
Ingredients:
Chicken breast chunks
Bell peppers, onions, cherry tomatoes
Olive oil, garlic, rosemary

**Preparation:**
Marinate chicken in olive oil, garlic, and rosemary.
Thread chicken and vegetables onto skewers, grill until cooked.

Prep Time: 30 minutes
GI Value: N/A
GI Load: N/A
Carbohydrates: 10g per skewer
Sugar: 4g
Calories: 200

Day 14:

Quinoa and Black Bean Bowl
Ingredients:
Cooked quinoa
Black beans, corn, avocado
Lime, cilantro, salt, and pepper

**Preparation:**
Mix quinoa with black beans, corn, and diced avocado.
Squeeze lime, add cilantro, and season with salt and
pepper.
Prep Time: 20 minutes
GI Value: 53
GI Load: 13
Carbohydrates: 30g per serving
Sugar: 1g
Calories: 220

Day 15:
Roasted Vegetable Frittata
Ingredients:
Eggs
Mixed vegetables (zucchini, bell peppers, cherry tomatoes)
Feta cheese, herbs

**Preparation:**
Roast vegetables in the oven.
Whisk eggs, pour over vegetables, top with feta and herbs, and bake.
Prep Time: 30 minutes
GI Value: N/A
GI Load: N/A
Carbohydrates: 8g per serving
Sugar: 4g
Calories: 220

Day 16:
Turkey and Quinoa Stuffed Peppers
Ingredients:
Ground turkey
Quinoa, black beans, corn
Taco seasoning, cheese

**Preparation:**
Cook turkey with taco seasoning.
Mix with quinoa, black beans, and corn. Stuff into peppers
and bake.
Prep Time: 35 minutes
GI Value: N/A
GI Load: N/A
Carbohydrates: 15g per serving
Sugar: 5g
Calories: 250

Day 17:
Zoodle Stir-Fry with Shrimp
Ingredients:
Zucchini noodles
Shrimp, broccoli, snap peas
Soy sauce, garlic, ginger

**Preparation:**
Sauté shrimp, broccoli, and snap peas with garlic and
ginger.
Add zucchini noodles and soy sauce, stir-fry until cooked.
Prep Time: 25 minutes
GI Value: N/A
GI Load: N/A
Carbohydrates: 10g per serving
Sugar: 3g
Calories: 200

Day 18:

Chicken and Vegetable Curry
Ingredients:
Chicken breast
Mixed vegetables (cauliflower, peas, carrots)
Curry sauce, coconut milk

**Preparation:**
Sauté chicken, add mixed vegetables, curry sauce, and coconut milk.
Simmer until chicken is cooked and vegetables are tender.
Prep Time: 40 minutes
GI Value: N/A
GI Load: N/A
Carbohydrates: 15g per serving
Sugar: 5g
Calories: 250

Day 19:

Spinach and Mushroom Omelette
Ingredients:
Eggs
Spinach, mushrooms, onions
Feta cheese, herbs

**Preparation:**
Sauté mushrooms and onions, add spinach until wilted.
Pour whisked eggs over, cook until set, and fold in half.
Top with feta and herbs.

Prep Time: 20 minutes
GI Value: N/A
GI Load: N/A
Carbohydrates: 8g per serving
Sugar: 2g
Calories: 180


## Day 20:

Baked Sweet Potato Fries
Ingredients:
Sweet potatoes
Olive oil, paprika, garlic powder

**Preparation:**
Cut sweet potatoes into fries.
Toss with olive oil, paprika, and garlic powder. Bake until crispy.
Prep Time: 30 minutes
GI Value: 63
GI Load: 17
Carbohydrates: 30g per serving
Sugar: 6g
Calories: 220

Day 21:
Shrimp and Avocado Salad
Ingredients:
Shrimp
Mixed greens, cherry tomatoes, avocado
Olive oil, lemon juice, salt, and pepper

**Preparation:**
Grill or sauté shrimp.
Toss with mixed greens, cherry tomatoes, and diced avocado. Dress with olive oil, lemon juice, salt, and pepper.
Prep Time: 15 minutes
GI Value: N/A
GI Load: N/A
Carbohydrates: 15g per serving
Sugar: 2g
Calories: 180

Day 22:
Quinoa and Vegetable Stir-Fry
Ingredients:
Cooked quinoa
Mixed vegetables (broccoli, carrots, snap peas)
Soy sauce, garlic, ginger

**Preparation:**
Sauté mixed vegetables with garlic and ginger.
Add cooked quinoa and soy sauce, stir-fry until heated through.
Prep Time: 20 minutes
GI Value: 53
GI Load: 13
Carbohydrates: 30g per serving
Sugar: 1g
Calories: 220

## Day 23:

Baked Chicken with Rosemary and Lemon
Ingredients:
Chicken thighs
Rosemary, lemon, garlic

**Preparation:**
Season chicken with rosemary, lemon juice, and minced garlic.
Bake until chicken is golden and cooked through.
Prep Time: 35 minutes
GI Value: N/A
GI Load: N/A
Carbohydrates: 0g
Sugar: 0g
Calories: 250

Day 24:
Black Bean and Corn Salad
Ingredients:
Black beans, corn, avocado
Red onion, cilantro, lime

**Preparation:**
Mix black beans, corn, diced avocado, red onion, and cilantro.
Squeeze lime over the salad and toss.
Prep Time: 15 minutes
GI Value: 41
GI Load: 6
Carbohydrates: 20g per serving
Sugar: 2g
Calories: 200


Day 25:
Grilled Eggplant and Tomato Sandwich
Ingredients:
Eggplant slices
Tomato slices, mozzarella
Whole grain bread, pesto

**Preparation:**
Grill eggplant slices.
Assemble sandwiches with eggplant, tomato, mozzarella, and a spread of pesto.
Prep Time: 25 minutes

GI Value: N/A
GI Load: N/A
Carbohydrates: 30g per sandwich
Sugar: 5g
Calories: 250

## Day 26:

Turkey and Vegetable Skillet
Ingredients:
Ground turkey
Mixed vegetables (bell peppers, zucchini, onions)
Taco seasoning, salsa

**Preparation:**
Cook turkey with taco seasoning.
Add mixed vegetables and salsa, cook until vegetables are tender.
Prep Time: 30 minutes
GI Value: N/A
GI Load: N/A
Carbohydrates: 15g per serving
Sugar: 5g
Calories: 250

Day 27:
Spaghetti Squash with Marinara Sauce
Ingredients:
Spaghetti squash
Marinara sauce, garlic, basil

**Preparation:**
Roast spaghetti squash until tender.
Scrape the flesh into strands, top with marinara sauce, garlic, and basil.
Prep Time: 45 minutes
GI Value: 40
GI Load: 7
Carbohydrates: 15g per serving
Sugar: 5g
Calories: 180


Day 28:
Chicken and Avocado Wrap
Ingredients:
Grilled chicken strips
Whole grain wrap, avocado
Lettuce, tomato, Greek yogurt

**Preparation:**
Grill chicken strips.
Assemble wraps with chicken, avocado, lettuce, tomato, and a dollop of Greek yogurt.
Prep Time: 20 minutes

GI Value: N/A
GI Load: N/A
Carbohydrates: 30g per wrap
Sugar: 5g
Calories: 250

## Day 29:

Quinoa and Black Bean Stuffed Peppers
Ingredients:
Cooked quinoa
Black beans, corn, tomatoes
Taco seasoning, cheese

**Preparation:**
Mix quinoa with black beans, corn, and diced tomatoes.
Stuff bell peppers, sprinkle with taco seasoning and cheese, and bake.
Prep Time: 35 minutes
GI Value: 53
GI Load: 13
Carbohydrates: 30g per serving
Sugar: 1g
Calories: 220

Day 30:
Salmon and Asparagus Foil Pack
Ingredients:
Salmon fillets
Asparagus spears
Lemon, garlic, dill

**Preparation:**
Place salmon and asparagus on a foil sheet.
Season with lemon, garlic, and dill. Seal and bake.
Prep Time: 30 minutes
GI Value: N/A
GI Load: N/A
Carbohydrates: 5g per serving
Sugar: 2g
Calories: 250

Day 31:
Lentil and Sweet Potato Soup
Ingredients:
Lentils
Sweet potatoes, carrots, celery
Vegetable broth, cumin, paprika

**Preparation:**
Cook lentils and set aside.
Sauté sweet potatoes, carrots, and celery in vegetable broth, add cumin and paprika. Mix in lentils and simmer.
Prep Time: 40 minutes

GI Value: 29
GI Load: 5
Carbohydrates: 20g per serving
Sugar: 2g
Calories: 200


## Day 32:

Greek Yogurt Parfait with Berries
Ingredients:
Greek yogurt
Mixed berries
Granola, honey

**Preparation:**
Layer Greek yogurt with mixed berries and granola.
Drizzle with honey.
Prep Time: 10 minutes
GI Value: N/A
GI Load: N/A
Carbohydrates: 15g per serving
Sugar: 10g
Calories: 180


## Day 33:

Turkey and Vegetable Lettuce Wraps
Ingredients:
Ground turkey
Lettuce leaves
Mixed vegetables (bell peppers, onions, water chestnuts)

**Preparation:**
Cook ground turkey with mixed vegetables.
Spoon into lettuce leaves to create wraps.
Prep Time: 25 minutes
GI Value: N/A
GI Load: N/A
Carbohydrates: 10g per serving
Sugar: 4g
Calories: 200

## Day 34:

Chickpea and Spinach Curry
Ingredients:
Chickpeas
Fresh spinach, tomatoes
Curry sauce, coconut milk

**Preparation:**
Sauté chickpeas with fresh spinach and tomatoes.
Add curry sauce and coconut milk, simmer until flavors meld.
Prep Time: 30 minutes
GI Value: N/A
GI Load: N/A
Carbohydrates: 15g per serving
Sugar: 5g
Calories: 250

## Day 35:

Egg and Vegetable Muffin Cups
Ingredients:
Eggs
Mixed vegetables (spinach, tomatoes, bell peppers)
Feta cheese, herbs

**Preparation:**
Whisk eggs and mix with chopped vegetables and herbs.
Pour into muffin cups, top with feta, and bake until set.
Prep Time: 25 minutes
GI Value: N/A
GI Load: N/A
Carbohydrates: 8g per serving
Sugar: 4g
Calories: 220

## Day 36:

Turkey and Quinoa Meatballs
Ingredients:
Ground turkey
Cooked quinoa
Marinara sauce, garlic, oregano

**Preparation:**
Mix ground turkey with cooked quinoa, garlic, and oregano.
Form into meatballs, bake and serve with marinara sauce.
Prep Time: 35 minutes

GI Value: N/A
GI Load: N/A
Carbohydrates: 15g per serving
Sugar: 5g
Calories: 250


## Day 37:

Cauliflower and Broccoli Gratin
Ingredients:
Cauliflower florets
Broccoli florets
Cheese sauce, breadcrumbs

**Preparation:**
Steam cauliflower and broccoli until tender.
Layer in a baking dish, pour cheese sauce, top with breadcrumbs, and bake until golden.
Prep Time: 30 minutes
GI Value: N/A
GI Load: N/A
Carbohydrates: 15g per serving
Sugar: 5g
Calories: 200

Day 38:

Shrimp and Quinoa Salad
Ingredients:
Quinoa
Shrimp, cherry tomatoes, cucumber
Lemon, olive oil, salt, and pepper

**Preparation:**
Cook quinoa and let it cool.
Mix with grilled shrimp, cherry tomatoes, and cucumber.
Dress with lemon, olive oil, salt, and pepper.
Prep Time: 25 minutes
GI Value: 53
GI Load: 13
Carbohydrates: 30g per serving
Sugar: 1g
Calories: 220


Day 39:

Zucchini Noodles with Pesto
Ingredients:
Zucchini noodles
Cherry tomatoes, pine nuts
Pesto sauce

**Preparation:**
Sauté zucchini noodles, cherry tomatoes, and pine nuts.
Toss with pesto sauce.
Prep Time: 15 minutes

GI Value: N/A
GI Load: N/A
Carbohydrates: 10g per serving
Sugar: 4g
Calories: 180


## Day 40:

Chicken and Vegetable Skewers
Ingredients:
Chicken breast chunks
Bell peppers, onions, cherry tomatoes
Olive oil, garlic, rosemary

**Preparation:**
Marinate chicken in olive oil, garlic, and rosemary.
Thread chicken and vegetables onto skewers, grill until cooked.
Prep Time: 30 minutes
GI Value: N/A
GI Load: N/A
Carbohydrates: 10g per skewer
Sugar: 4g
Calories: 200


## Day 41:

Quinoa and Black Bean Bowl
Ingredients:
Cooked quinoa
Black beans, corn, avocado

Lime, cilantro, salt, and pepper

**Preparation:**
Mix quinoa with black beans, corn, and diced avocado.
Squeeze lime, add cilantro, and season with salt and pepper.
Prep Time: 20 minutes
GI Value: 53
GI Load: 13
Carbohydrates: 30g per serving
Sugar: 1g
Calories: 220

## Day 42:

Grilled Vegetable Wrap
Ingredients:
Grilled vegetables (zucchini, eggplant, bell peppers)
Whole grain wrap, hummus
Spinach, feta cheese

**Preparation:**
Grill vegetables until tender.
Assemble wraps with grilled vegetables, hummus, spinach, and crumbled feta.
Prep Time: 25 minutes
GI Value: N/A
GI Load: N/A
Carbohydrates: 30g per wrap
Sugar: 5g
Calories: 250

Day 43:
Lentil and Vegetable Stew
Ingredients:
1 cup lentils
Mixed vegetables (carrots, celery, onions)
Vegetable broth, garlic, cumin, coriander

**Preparation:**
Cook lentils and set aside.
Sauté vegetables in garlic, add cumin and coriander.
Mix in lentils and vegetable broth.
Prep Time: 30 minutes
GI Value: 29
GI Load: 5
Carbohydrates: 20g per serving
Sugar: 2g
Calories: 200

Day 44:
Greek Chicken Salad
Ingredients:
Grilled chicken breast
Mixed greens, cherry tomatoes, cucumber
Feta cheese, olives

**Preparation:**
Grill chicken and slice into strips.
Combine with mixed greens, cherry tomatoes, cucumber,
feta, and olives.

Prep Time: 20 minutes
GI Value: N/A
GI Load: N/A
Carbohydrates: 15g per serving
Sugar: 3g
Calories: 180


## Day 45:

Chia Seed Pudding with Berries
Ingredients:
Chia seeds
Almond milk
Mixed berries
Honey for sweetness

**Preparation:**
Mix chia seeds and almond milk, refrigerate overnight.
Top with mixed berries and a drizzle of honey.
Prep Time: 10 minutes (+overnight chilling)
GI Value: 1
GI Load: 0
Carbohydrates: 15g per serving
Sugar: 0g
Calories: 120

# Comprehensive groceries list

A shopping list for a Glycemic Index (GI) diet involves selecting a variety of foods with different GI values to ensure a balanced and health-conscious approach. Below is a detailed shopping list categorized by food groups, including their GI values and Glycemic Load (GL) counters:

**Fruits:**
2. Apples (GI: 36, GL: 5)
3. Berries (strawberries, blueberries, raspberries) (GI: 40-53, GL: 5-8)
4. Pears (GI: 38, GL: 4)
5. Cherries (GI: 22, GL: 3)
6. Grapes (GI: 46, GL: 11)
7. Oranges (GI: 40, GL: 5)
8. Kiwi (GI: 53, GL: 7)
9. Plums (GI: 39, GL: 5)
10. Peaches (GI: 42, GL: 5)
11. Watermelon (GI: 76, GL: 8) (for occasional consumption)

**Vegetables:**
1. Broccoli (GI: 10, GL: 1)
2. Spinach (GI: 6, GL: 0)
3. Tomatoes (GI: 15, GL: 2)
4. Carrots (GI: 41, GL: 5)
5. Sweet potatoes (GI: 44, GL: 11)
6. Zucchini (GI: 15, GL: 2)

7. Bell peppers (GI: 10, GL: 1)
8. Cauliflower (GI: 15, GL: 2)
9. Asparagus (GI: 15, GL: 2)
10. Cabbage (GI: 10, GL: 1)

## Grains:

1. Quinoa (GI: 53, GL: 13)
2. Brown rice (GI: 50, GL: 16)
3. Barley (GI: 28, GL: 6)
4. Buckwheat (GI: 54, GL: 10)
5. Whole grain oats (GI: 55, GL: 13)
6. Whole wheat pasta (GI: 37, GL: 10)
7. Bulgur (GI: 48, GL: 12)
8. Couscous (GI: 65, GL: 9) (moderate use)

## Proteins:

1. Chicken breast (unprocessed)
2. Salmon (fresh)
3. Tofu
4. Lentils (GI: 29, GL: 5)
5. Chickpeas (GI: 28, GL: 9)
6. Black beans (GI: 30, GL: 7)

## Eggs

1. Greek yogurt (unsweetened) (GI: 11, GL: 3)

## Dairy:

2. Low-fat milk (GI: 31, GL: 5)
3. Cheese (moderate use)
4. Cottage cheese (GI: 10, GL: 3)

5. Plain yogurt (unsweetened) (GI: 14, GL: 4)

**Nuts and Seeds:**
1. Almonds (GI: 0, GL: 0)
2. Walnuts (GI: 0, GL: 0)
3. Chia seeds (GI: 1, GL: 0)
4. Flaxseeds (GI: 1, GL: 0)
5. Sunflower seeds (GI: 1, GL: 0)

**Oils and Fats:**
1. Olive oil (GI: 0, GL: 0)
2. Avocado (GI: 15, GL: 1)
3. Coconut oil (for cooking in moderation)
4. Butter (moderate use)

**Beverages:**
1. Water
2. Herbal teas (unsweetened)
3. Green tea (unsweetened)
4. Coffee (black or with minimal added sugar)

**Condiments:**
1. Mustard
2. Vinegar
3. Herbs and spices (e.g., cinnamon, turmeric, oregano)
4. Soy sauce (low sodium)
5. Tomato sauce (unsweetened) (moderate use)

**Sweeteners (Use sparingly):**
1. Honey (GI: 58, GL: 12)
2. Maple syrup (GI: 54, GL: 12)
3. Snacks (Occasional):
4. Dark chocolate (70% cocoa or higher) (GI: 23, GL: 6)
5. Popcorn (GI: 65, GL: 12) (air-popped, without added butter or sugar)

**Miscellaneous:**
1. Whole grain bread (GI: 49, GL: 11)
2. Whole grain crackers (GI: 67, GL: 10) (moderate use)
3. Salsa (unsweetened)
4. Olives

**Frozen Foods (Moderate Use):**
1. Frozen vegetables (e.g., broccoli, spinach)
2. Frozen berries (unsweetened)

**Prepared Foods (Read Labels):**
1. Prepared soups (low sodium, check labels for added sugars)
2. Prepared salads (check dressings for added sugars)
3. Meat Alternatives:
4. Plant-based protein sources (e.g., Beyond Meat, tofu-based products)

**Gluten-Free Options:**

1. Gluten-free oats
2. Quinoa pasta
3. Brown rice pasta
4. Considerations for Moderation:
5. Potatoes (GI: 50, GL: 18)
6. White rice (GI: 73, GL: 28)
7. Bananas (GI: 51, GL: 12)
8. Dried fruits (moderate use, check labels for added sugars)

## Tips for Smart Shopping:

1. Read labels for added sugars and processing levels.
2. Choose fresh, whole foods over processed alternatives.
3. Shop the perimeter of the grocery store for fresh produce and unprocessed items.
4. Buy in bulk when possible to save money on staples.
5. Be mindful of portion sizes and adjust quantities based on your needs.

In the journey towards optimal health and well-being, understanding the impact of our dietary choices is paramount. The exploration of Glycemic Index (GI) diets and Glycemic Load (GL) counters has been a transformative guide, illuminating the intricate relationship between food, blood sugar levels, and overall health.

Throughout this comprehensive guide, we've delved into the intricacies of the Glycemic Index, unraveling its significance in deciphering the carbohydrate content of various foods. From the basics of what the Glycemic Index entails to its crucial role in managing conditions such as diabetes and aiding in weight management, our exploration has been both enlightening and empowering.

The journey began by demystifying the Glycemic Index itself—shedding light on how different carbohydrates impact blood sugar levels. We explored the physiological processes governing digestion, blood sugar regulation, and carbohydrate metabolism, providing a foundation for understanding the intricacies of the GI concept.

As we navigated further, the guide unfolded the practical application of the Glycemic Index in real-life scenarios. From managing diabetes to leveraging the Glycemic Load for nuanced decision-making in meal planning, each section aimed at empowering readers to make informed, health-conscious choices.

The journey extended beyond theory to practical implementation, offering a wealth of knowledge on crafting low-GI meal plans, understanding Glycemic Load, and making food choices that align with personal health goals. We delved into the world of low-GI foods, exploring diverse categories, including fruits, vegetables, proteins, and even desserts, all while providing detailed nutritional information for each.

The guide also presented a 45-day meal plan, meticulously curated to offer a diverse range of low-GI recipes, ensuring not only health benefits but also a delightful culinary experience. From breakfast to dinner, each recipe was crafted with a holistic understanding of the Glycemic Index, providing readers with a roadmap for sustained, health-conscious eating.

In essence, this guide is a compass for those seeking to navigate the complex landscape of nutrition with precision. It stands as a testament to the transformative power of informed dietary choices, reminding us that what we eat plays a pivotal role in shaping our health and vitality.

As you embark on your journey towards a healthier, more conscious way of eating, may this guide serve as a trusted companion—a beacon of knowledge illuminating the path to optimal well-being through the prism of the Glycemic Index and Glycemic Load Counters. Here's to a healthier, happier you

Dear Esteemed Customer,

I hope this book has been a source of inspiration, comfort, and profound insights for you. Each recipe was crafted with care, meticulous attention to detail, and a deep understanding of how to effectively utilize the comprehensive guide to glycemic index diet, ensuring the creation of wholesome and nutritious meals. Your reviews, experiences, and insights are truly invaluable to me.

Every assessment motivates me to refine and tailor my work to better meet your needs. Let's foster a meaningful dialogue—a conversation that goes beyond the written words, building a stronger connection. Your thoughts serve as the driving force behind our continuous journey of improvement.

Warm Regards,

*Luisa pace*